Praise for *Inside the Minds*

"What C-Level executives read to keep their edge and make pivotal business decisions. Timeless classics for indispensable knowledge." - Richard Costello, Manager-Corporate Marketing Communication, General Electric (NYSE: GE)

"Want to know what the real leaders are thinking about now? It's in here." - Carl Ledbetter, SVP & CTO, Novell, Inc.

"Priceless wisdom from experts at applying technology in support of business objectives." - Frank Campagnoni, CTO, GE Global Exchange Services

"Unique insights into the way the experts think and the lessons they've learned from experience." - MT Rainey, Co-CEO, Young & Rubicam/Rainey Kelly Campbell Roalfe

"Unlike any other business book." - Bruce Keller, Partner, Debevoise & Plimpton

"The Inside the Minds series is a valuable probe into the thought, perspectives, and techniques of accomplished professionals. By taking a 50,000 foot view, the authors place their endeavors in a context rarely gleaned from text books or treatise." - Chuck Birenbaum, Partner, Thelen Reid & Priest

"A must read for anyone in the industry." - Dr. Chuck Lucier, Chief Growth Officer, Booz-Allen & Hamilton

"A must read for those who manage at the intersection of business and technology." - Frank Roney, General Manager, IBM

"A great way to see across the changing marketing landscape at a time of significant innovation." - David Kenny, Chairman & CEO, Digitas

"An incredible resource of information to help you develop outside-the-box..." - Rich Jernstedt, CEO, Golin/Harris International

"A snapshot of everything you need..." - Charles Koob, Co-Head of Litigation Department, Simpson Thacher & Bartlet

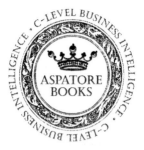

www.Aspatore.com

Aspatore Books is the largest and most exclusive publisher of C-Level executives (CEO, CFO, CTO, CMO, Partner) from the world's most respected companies. Aspatore annually publishes C-Level executives from over half the Global 500, top 250 professional services firms, law firms (MPs/Chairs), and other leading companies of all sizes. By focusing on publishing only C-Level executives, Aspatore provides professionals of all levels with proven business intelligence from industry insiders, rather than relying on the knowledge of unknown authors and analysts. Aspatore Books is committed to publishing a highly innovative line of business books, redefining and expanding the meaning of such books as indispensable resources for professionals of all levels. In addition to individual best-selling business titles, Aspatore Books publishes the following unique lines of business books: Inside the Minds, Business Bibles, Bigwig Briefs, C-Level Business Review (Quarterly), Book Binders, ExecRecs, and The C-Level Test, innovative resources for all professionals. Aspatore is a privately held company headquartered in Boston, Massachusetts, with employees around the world.

Inside the Minds

The critically acclaimed *Inside the Minds* series provides readers of all levels with proven business intelligence from C-Level executives (CEO, CFO, CTO, CMO, Partner) from the world's most respected companies. Each chapter is comparable to a white paper or essay and is a future-oriented look at where an industry/profession/topic is heading and the most important issues for future success. Each author has been carefully chosen through an exhaustive selection process by the *Inside the Minds* editorial board to write a chapter for this book. *Inside the Minds* was conceived in order to give readers actual insights into the leading minds of business executives worldwide. Because so few books or other publications are actually written by executives in industry, *Inside the Minds* presents an unprecedented look at various industries and professions never before available.

Inside the Minds:
The Art & Science of Plastic Surgery

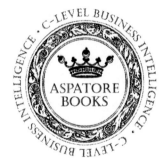

If you are a C-Level executive interested in submitting a manuscript to the Aspatore editorial board, please email jason@aspatore.com. Include your book idea, your biography, and any additional pertinent information.

Published by Aspatore, Inc.

For corrections, company/title updates, comments or any other inquiries please email info@aspatore.com.

First Printing, 2004
10 9 8 7 6 5 4 3 2 1

ISBN 1-58762-278-5 Library of Congress Control Number: 2004102574

Inside the Minds Managing Editor, Laura Kearns, Edited by Michaela Falls, Proofread by Eddie Fournier, Cover design by Scott Rattray & Ian Mazie

Inside the Minds:
The Art & Science of Plastic Surgery

CONTENTS

Court Cutting, M.D.   7
PRACTICING THE CRAFT OF PLASTIC
SURGERY

Craig R. Dufresne, M.D., FACS   25
THE MARRIAGE OF ART & SURGERY –
SURGERY & ART

Barry J. Cohen, M.D., FACS   43
THE REWARDS OF PLASTIC SURGERY

Jay M. Pensler, M.D.   65
PLASTIC SURGERY FOR A NEW
MILLENNIUM

Lance G. Leithauser, M.D.   75
THE SUCCESSFUL PLASTIC SURGEON

A. Dean Jabs, M.D., Ph.D., FACS &   83
Franklin D. Richards, M.D., FACS
FOCUSING ON THE PATIENT

Mark E. Richards, M.D.   97
*UNDERSTANDING THE AESTHETIC PLASTIC
SURGEON*

Louis P. Bucky, M.D., FACS   115
THE ABCS OF PLASTIC SURGERY

Michael Olding, M.D., FACS   125
COMMUNICATING WITH THE PATIENT

David T.W. Chiu, M.D., FACS, FAAP   135
ENVISIONING THE END RESULT

Amitabha Mitra, M.D., FACS   147
THE EVOLUTION OF PLASTIC SURGERY

Khosrow Matini, M.D., FACS   163
*PLASTIC SURGERY AND PLASTIC SURGEONS
IN THE 21ST CENTURY*

Appendix   181
*BODY CONTOURING FOLLOWING
BARIATRIC SURGERY*

Practicing the Craft of Plastic Surgery

Court Cutting, M.D.

Director, Cleft Lip and Palate Program
Institute of Reconstructive Plastic Surgery
New York University Medical Center

Not an Art, Not a Science – a Craft

Plastic surgery is not a true art, but more of a craft. Picasso made things no one else had seen before. Plastic surgery does not have that luxury – we are practicing a craft. We do the same things over and over. We have a mental picture of the average beautiful face, for example, that we try to bring patients into. We don't have the freedom to do a Jackson Pollock on somebody's face. It's certainly a very interesting craft and a difficult one.

The tools we use to work in this craft have to be based on surgical science. The human body is actually a terrible art medium: It needs blood supply to stay alive; it scars; it grows – all problems the average artist or craftsperson doesn't have to deal with when they're working in their medium. From medical science, and particularly surgical science, we know how wounds will heal and how they will contract, and we have some idea of how a face will grow, particularly in response to the surgical trauma we inflict. These are all important considerations. They represent the palettes the plastic surgeon uses to achieve his or her ends.

One of the oddities you'll notice about a plastic surgeon is we claim no particular organ system. A urologist works on the kidneys and the urinary system; a cardiac surgeon works on the heart; but the plastic surgeon seems to be all over the place. We do breast surgery, hand surgery; I do a lot of facial reconstruction surgery. So why does a plastic surgeon work all over the body?

The reason is that plastic surgeons might be defined as surgical problem solvers. Whenever a problem crops up with a patient that doesn't seem to fit into anyone else's discipline, and somehow needs a surgeon, it becomes a plastic surgery problem. That's how plastic surgery became what it is and why we are all over the body. We tend to use surgical principles to solve problems that you can't find preconceived surgical answers for.

In terms of the qualities a plastic surgeon needs to have, probably the most important is to be a doctor, to care about your patients and hold their needs first in your mind. Ethics are absolutely critical. I see in plastic surgeons today the tendency to go from doctor to salesman. Many of the young plastic surgeons are so anxious to get their practice built. It's almost as if they're selling cosmetics at a department store counter. Furthering their own ends becomes more important than being sure a particular procedure is best for the patient. It's something young plastic surgeons need to fight. It will kill your practice in the long run. Your patients need to know that you care about them and that you want to make them better rather than making the payments on your new sports car.

Communication: Listen to the Voices that Matter Most

Communicating with patients should be done one-on-one with them. Although occasionally we must use phone calls or emails, most of time it should be face-to-face. One way you should *not* communicate with your patients is by hiring a publicist. The idea of mass marketing a particular doctor to a patient without knowing what that particular patient wants or needs truly scares me, although it's prevalent throughout the industry. You see plastic surgeons advertising on billboards. This is not how you communicate with patients.

Of course, with a neonate or a child in the preverbal stage, you actually communicate with their parents, and you continue doing that until they're 18 years old. I have a breakpoint when I take care of children. I try assiduously to avoid operating on kids in the "terrible twos." They are in a very difficult period when they try to reject everything external. In the first year of life through 18 months, the parents have total control, and their child will have what the parents want and often what the doctor wants. But after that, I try to leave the kids alone as much as possible and let them begin to express their own needs and wants as to when a particular surgery will occur.

I see parents of a three-year-old with a cleft lip who had surgery done at another institution that didn't come out perfect, but it's not terrible. These parents want me to fix it, but the child sees nothing wrong – the kid thinks it's fine. You don't want to operate for the parents; you want to operate for the child. The situation comes up again very frequently in the teenage years. The parent wants the child to have *x, y,* or *z* procedure, but the child needs a break: Learning to listen to both of those voices – the child's voice and that of the parents – can sometimes be very challenging.

In a situation like that, I usually go with the child's desires. If the parent wants the child to have surgery the child doesn't want, for me the child wins – unless the child is very young and can't know the implications of such a decision. Then, of course, the parents make the decision, and the surgery happens.

To make that child feel more comfortable, ethics demand that you make sure the family knows you are trying to do the best thing for the child, rather than for yourself. The situation boils down to trust in the end. The parents need to feel very comfortable that they are in the right place and that we are all trying to do the right thing.

The Initial Visit – in the Womb

It's interesting how an initial visit before surgery has changed over the years. I used to have patients with cleft lip and palate referred by their pediatricians. Now I see them prenatally referred by the obstetrician. Ultrasound has changed everything.

Our kids are often diagnosed before birth, and I begin the interaction with the parents then. I try not to be judgmental in any way, obviously. I know this disease can be very well treated and the kids do fine, but I never insert myself into the abortion debate. That's none of my business, and it's a difficult enough decision for parents when they have to make it.

In my entire practice, I've had only three sets of parents actually decide to abort after they see how other kids have done and after they've talked to other parents. I imagine that number is low because I have a selected population: I'm seeing parents who have already decided to at least consider having the baby. That's how my relationship with them starts. The disorder occurs usually between the eighth week and the tenth week of the pregnancy, but usually within about a month, ultrasound will provide a fairly clear idea of how things will look.

Before ultrasound, when a baby was born with a cleft lip or palate, it was a complete shock to everyone. Often the obstetrician had never seen a baby with this deformity. I remember one birth in particular: The obstetrician saw the baby, gasped, threw a blanket over the child's face, and whisked him off to the nurse. The family had no knowledge base that the problem could be taken care of, and everyone was thrown into a major depression.

With prenatal diagnosis via ultrasound, the approach is altogether different. Well before the baby is born, the parents have the entire course of treatment laid out for their child – exactly what they can expect. This early knowledge has changed everything for the better. The family is perfectly comfortable. They know the child will be born with a cleft; they know what to expect with treatment; and they know everything will turn out fine. Beginning in that neonatal period, we work with the parents, taking one step at a time, and then, as the patient progresses through childhood, our relationship becomes more typically doctor-patient.

There have been other changes, as well, particularly relative to the cleft lip and palate patient.

When I was trying to get my practice started in New York some 20 years ago, I called my old professor and said, "Dr. Bardach, how will I get my practice going? There are nearly 20 different cleft palate centers in New York?" He told me not to worry – if I get 20 patients in the beginning, they will be my practice for the life of my practice. And he would have been right because, back then, we operated on the same kids over and over. These days, with the techniques we've developed here at the Institute, with the orthodontist and the prosthodontist I work with, the surgeries are usually completed by the end of the baby's first year of life. And if everything has gone well, I don't operate on them again until their mid-teens, when it's time for a little touchup on the nose.

I love second opinions. Most doctors don't like them – I think because they're afraid they'll lose those patients. I feel exactly the opposite. I have a group of people around the country about whom I feel very confident and who do a wonderful job at what I do. If parents feel unsure about a procedure or unhappy with a particular outcome, I encourage them to get second opinions from any of those people. Any doctor who doesn't want a parent to seek a second opinion is insecure.

Cosmetic versus Reconstructive Surgery

I believe there should be no difference in the way you treat a cosmetic patient versus the way you treat a reconstructive patient. I know that's an outlier point of view. When a patient comes to you with a problem or a complaint, you are still a doctor, regardless of the complaint, and you should address the complaint as a doctor.

The reconstructive patient often has more realistic expectations than the cosmetic patient. Sometimes the cosmetic patient has a feeling that they will go from age 70 to age 25 again, and the unethical practitioner promotes and sells the snake oil, playing on that false hope. These patients may look better, but they don't get what they wanted.

Cosmetic surgery can be awesome. Some of the happiest patients I have are cosmetic patients. But you must let them know the risks and benefits of the procedure – and promote realistic expectations. And, again, you approach them as you would a reconstructive patient: Help them have their feet set solidly on the ground when they go into surgery.

Innovation is Critical

It is absolutely essential to be innovative as a plastic surgeon. I certainly wouldn't be where I am if I weren't. The quality that distinguishes a plastic surgeon is his ability as a problem solver, and that demands innovation. If you don't innovate, you'll wind up in the back of the pack.

We have a tremendous number of professional meetings at which we speak and in which we participate every year. The sheer number would be burdensome if the meetings were not always so very helpful. We also read and contribute to medical journals.

Being actively involved in research is extremely helpful. As a surgical problem-solver, the plastic surgeon has his palette of procedures, but when he knows a procedure in common practice doesn't work, or when he hits a wall with a difficult problem, he must go to the bench or to the research lab to solve it; otherwise, I don't know how he'd be able to get up in the morning. Participating in research and learning some of the innovations that will come along before they are in standard practice are invaluable.

Surgery will be revolutionized when we understand fetal wound healing. A pediatric surgeon, Dr. Michael Harrison in San Francisco, began operating on fetuses for problems that were incompatible with life after delivery. This surgery is not something you undertake lightly – there are often spontaneous miscarriages following these procedures. But for some life-threatening problems, the results are outstanding.

One of the discoveries is that fetuses heal without scarring, at least in the first half of pregnancy. They heal regeneratively, like a shellfish that loses a claw and generates a new claw. If a human loses a hand, we put a scar cap over the end of it. Somewhere in evolution our bodies learned that scarring is quicker than regeneration, and we picked up that ability as time went on. But early in our embryogenesis, we retain that regenerative healing that is common with lower life forms. Once we figure out how we can turn off scarring and go back to regenerative healing, surgery will be changed forever. Think of the possibilities: No scars anywhere, re-growing tissue you've lost when you need it back. How extraordinary it will be to learn how that happens.

When Experimental Surgery is Appropriate

There are certainly times when experimentation is absolutely essential. I see children with severe facial malformations that are one-of-a-kind, or that I might see once or twice in my entire practice. When this happens, you go to the books and find no standard recipe answer for how to care for these patients. In these situations, it is absolutely appropriate that experimental surgery be done.

You use your knowledge of surgical concepts and how the body responds to trauma to design a procedure that's unique to this specific patient in that singular situation. You must be open with the parents and the patient that you don't have a series of these surgeries behind you whose results you can share.

At other times, experimentation is inappropriate. There isn't a lot of room for experimentation in a facelift, for example. If you have an excellent answer for how to proceed with a facelift, and you are experimenting just to try to produce an article for self aggrandizement in a women's magazine, that experimentation is inadvisable. On the other hand, if the new procedure offers significant advantages over standard techniques, it should be approached carefully with the patient's eyes wide open.

Challenges and Rewards, Problems and Solutions

The most challenging aspect of being a plastic surgeon is the long hours. Additionally for me, because I care for kids all the time, I have the weight of the problems of hundreds of patients from birth to early adulthood that I carry with me all the time. I can never escape them – my patients are my patients from birth until they're 18 or 19 years old. Often their situations can leave me with a heavy heart due to the weight of all that parental worry.

My job is also incredibly satisfying and rewarding. The burdens and the rewards of being a plastic surgeon are intricately intertwined.

I measure success by the fact that I am working long days and operating all the time. But if you aren't careful, you discover you have left no time for your personal life. My wife would say I strike that balance poorly – I must admit that I'm a workaholic.

Imagination, intelligence, and ethics impress me in other plastic surgeons. If I see another plastic surgeon who exhibits those qualities, particularly if he or she is giving a presentation at a meeting with a wonderful idea I hadn't thought of or heard before, and yet I know that person is solid, I am impressed.

Being a leader in this field draws us back to innovation – careful, well considered innovation. The qualifications of "careful" and "well considered" are important. Surgeons who will innovate, or feel they are innovating, just to get their names in lights do not practice careful, well considered innovation. What they do is a gimmick to try to get their practice up above the pack. A plastic surgeon who innovates after careful thought to produce a real improvement over previously prescribed procedures is a leader in this field.

What I don't like personally is doing procedures where the problem has been solved long ago, and the solution works very well, and we continue to do the same thing over and over. Even in plastic surgery, we have our bread-and-butter cases, but doing very many of them time and again, day after day, can get tiring.

In other surgeons, I don't like those who see themselves as salespeople and to whom making payments on a Mercedes is more important than doing what their patients want or need. These surgeons disturb me greatly, and their numbers are increasing. Plastic surgery tends to attract the entrepreneurial among the medical students, and the results can be quite disgusting at times. At least, in plastic surgery, we have a peer review process, a board certification process that tries to keep these people from getting anywhere. But there are certainly many practitioners in allied specialties who do what is usually thought of as plastic surgical procedures where there is no such oversight. These people are all over the media, and their presence demeans our profession.

The best way for patients to avoid someone like this is through referrals. The best source of referrals is always a satisfied patient talking about his or her experience. That patient can tell another that there will be a scar after the surgery and that in the first six weeks, the wound will be thick and hard and red, but then it will get better in the next nine to 12 months. This veteran will show the potential patient the scar and share realities, so that when the patient comes to you, he or she knows what to expect, realistically. Referrals from other satisfied patients are by far the best.

Getting Real: Risks and Results

The biggest misconception among plastic surgery patients is that there will be no scar after surgery. Every time you cut, there is a scar.

People who expect the results of their procedure will be instant are not being realistic. Facelifts can be astonishing operations, for example, and I have had some incredibly satisfied facelift patients. But you are wounded. A facelift is a real operation. For about six months, you won't know how you're finally going to look. You might be presentable in three weeks, so you can get out and function again, but you will have a wound to heal, as in any other surgical procedure. You don't want to schedule a facelift two days – or even two months – before your daughter's wedding, and any plastic surgeon who tells you that you should does not have your best interest at heart.

The most common risks for plastic surgery patients are those of any other surgery: Anytime you get cut, you can bleed; you can get an infection. Most of the time, the risks of recipe surgical procedures are well described. You can look in the literature and read reports of a series of 500 appendectomies, where the complications associated with appendectomies are well described, and you can get those risks across to the patient. The same is true for many of the recipe surgical procedures we have in plastic surgery.

But in my practice, especially for a kid with facial malformations, I'm often developing a frankly experimental procedure tailored for this particular patient. So it's a little harder to foresee what the additional complications can be. In these cases, it's essential that the doctor and patient enter into a trust relationship and solve the problems together. If a complication occurs, it is essential that the doctor stay with the patient and solve the problem. This results in happy patients and fewer lawsuits.

I train scores of residents and surgical students. Some years ago, I got a piece of advice from a plastic surgeon in New York named Tom Rees as to how to build my practice. He told me that often your practice is built more by the patients you don't operate on than by the ones you do. Advising a patient that it's better not to have the surgery because what you can offer them won't get them where they want to go will often build your patient base faster than doing operations that won't work for those patients.

Right now, I'm emphasizing a very careful surgical technique that will help minimize scarring – gentleness. I'm always telling the residents that scars from stitch marks are caused by tying those loops of stitches too tightly, killing the tissue inside the stitches. Gentleness and treating the tissue with great respect produce the best results.

The Importance of Apprenticeship and Innovation

There is no substitute for apprenticeship. I was an R-10, which means I was trained as a resident for ten years after medical school and learned many different surgical skills from a multitude of great and talented people. People say to me that I'm a leader in the treatment of children with facial malformations, but if it seems that we see further than anyone else has seen before, it's because we stand on the shoulders of giants. I have several giants on whose shoulders I'm happy and proud to stand – Janusz Bardach, Joe McCarthy...I could go through a long list; I owe them so much.

I try to teach my students the same things that were taught me. They are an extension of me as they interact with patients, and I want them to behave with patients the same way I do. They should be professional, ethical, and helpful with the patient, even when the patients are sometimes hostile. Keep your cool and help them work through the problem.

Usually, it's innovation that separates the good surgeons from the great ones. There are some wonderful practitioners of plastic surgery who do the same procedures over and over. They do what they do extremely well, and that is a good plastic surgeon. There is nothing wrong with a doctor in a community private practice who does a very good job performing the recipe operations of plastic surgery. That is a commendable ability, and when I train a resident, that's the first thing I look for: a good, solid clinician.

But what elevates you above that level and into greatness is hitting a wall with a problem that the recipes don't solve – then, carefully and with much consideration, developing new ways to treat patients that take the specialty further. That difference makes a great plastic surgeon.

Merging Specialties for Dramatic Success

A most profound change is something that happened here at the Institute of Reconstructive Plastic Surgery at the New York University Medical Center. We have fortunately been funded by the National Foundation of Facial Rehabilitation so that we can pull together various forces that our kids, our patients, need for their care. One of the pleasures I've had is working with an incredible orthodontist, Barry Grayson.

When its founder first envisioned the Institute, he felt it was important to have an orthodontist and a speech therapist and other team members caring for our kids. What happened with this orthodontist is unique. We began to synthesize our specialties. The orthodontist began thinking like a surgeon, and the surgeon began thinking like an orthodontist.

For example, Dr. Grayson takes a newborn with a cleft lip and palate – very severe facial malformations – and spends the first three to four months of her life slowly molding her face, using the dimension of time. He applies small forces on her teeth and slowly, over some months, achieves a change. And now we've asked the orthodontist to pull himself out of teeth and reshape the entire nose and face. That, then, allows me to accomplish in one procedure what used to take three to four procedures over the child's first eight years of life. The results have been quite striking.

The same thing has happened with my associate, Joe McCarthy, who has learned to think like Dr. Grayson. We crack the bones in the face, and as the fracture is healing, slowly stretch the healing fracture to grow new bone and stretch the soft tissue, which is a foreign concept to a surgeon. Most surgeons think about how to solve a problem immediately. We're learning how to use the dimension of time, which is something the orthodontist is much more comfortable with.

Innovations: Virtual Surgery, Scarless Wounds

One of my research areas is 3-dimensional computer graphics. I do a lot of surgery in Third World countries trying to help kids in the developing world, particularly Vietnam, where I've been a number of times. There you'll see teenagers walking around on the streets with open, unrepaired cleft lips and palates, their lives devastated. I used to go there and do those surgeries, and after operating on 200 kids in two weeks, you felt good about yourself.

But you have to take a step back and really look at the problem. In China alone, there are 40,000 new cleft babies born every year. What I was doing was a drop in the bucket. The real answer is teaching local doctors how to care for this problem themselves.

The little ballet we've developed for solving the problem is like a complex 3D jigsaw puzzle you create yourself and then put together in a different way than when you started. It's very difficult to get the process across to the students. The 3D computer graphics have been helpful in defining these ideas and allowing us to transmit them to both the doctors in Third World countries and doctors in developed nations.

We have a few computer programs that help us do this. We began by developing animation tools. We use a 3D animation tool called Maya – it's very popular in Hollywood right now. We wrote some software in our lab that uses computer-animated models of kids with facial deformities to simulate patients. The student surgeons operate on these virtual patients and make their mistakes on them before they ever touch a live human. Its reality is almost scary.

For centuries surgeons have been trained by operating on the poor. The first time I took a knife to a patient, was it a child of a wealthy CEO living in Greenwich, Connecticut? No, it was on a child in a welfare hospital. Was I as good then as I am now? Of course not. Could I have made a mistake that that child would have paid for? Probably. Now, in the 21st century, I believe students should learn by operating on virtual patients and making their mistakes in the simulated environment before operating on a human.

A friend of mine who is an American Airlines pilot qualified on the 777 a couple of years ago, so I asked him what it was like to fly the 777. He said he didn't know what the actual plane felt like, that he had been trained on a simulator. They put him in a hurricane; he lost his landing gear; one of the engines flamed out; etc. He developed quick automatic responses to handle these emergency situations in a simulated environment, which he hopes he'll never experience in the real plane. But if he does, he'll know just how to handle it. I think that's what should happen with early surgical training.

We've been developing this program over the last four or five years, and we've seen that it has dramatically changed the way surgeons learn.

I keep hoping for that biochemical breakthrough I mentioned earlier that would allow a wound to heal with no scarring – developing drugs that help us control and manage wound healing, although some of the answer may lie in gene manipulation. I think that's where the big payoffs will be coming in the next ten to 20 years.

If you had a terrible scar on your arm, wouldn't it be great if you could just have it removed, and instead of a new scar in its place, your skin simply regenerated over the opening? It's incredible how that would revolutionize plastic surgery. We have the genetic information in our DNA to allow that kind of regeneration, but that gene has been turned off somewhere in our evolution. We have to figure out how to let it happen again.

Dr. Cutting obtained his M.D. from the University of Chicago in 1975. After a surgical internship at Yale University, he trained in otolaryngology and cleft lip and palate surgery at the University of Iowa. This was followed by a plastic surgery residency and craniofacial fellowship under Dr. Joseph McCarthy at New York University. During his training at NYU he extended Dr. McCarthy's NIH program grant into evaluation of craniofacial anomalies using computer graphic methods. For 16 years he has been funded by the NIH to study the statistical analysis of smoothly curving three-dimensional shape.

In 1992, Dr. Cutting traveled to Vietnam with Operation Smile to perform cleft lip and palate surgery. Five years ago Dr. Cutting began an affiliation with the Smile Train charity, which puts its entire focus on empowering the local surgeons in developing countries to solve their own cleft problem. Surgical education is the cornerstone of this effort. Using his knowledge of computer graphics, three-dimensional surgical animations and most recently a surgical simulation program were developed to facilitate teaching.

Dr. Cutting has been on the faculty at New York University for the past 20 years and is director of the Cleft Lip and Palate Program.

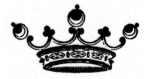

The Marriage of Art & Surgery – Surgery & Art

Craig R. Dufresne, M.D., FACS
Clinical Professor of Plastic Surgery
Georgetown University

Overview: Then and Now

The term "plastic surgery" was coined in the 19th century by German surgeons who used the term from the Greek which means to fold, mold and change shape. They used this term to describe how they would shape tissues into missing body parts and features. Plastic surgery has evolved much beyond that limited definition that is rooted in ancient history where surgery was designed to relieve facial deformity, in particular, amputations of the nose, ears and parts of the facial structure. The restoration of the individual, the person, was the goal.

The definition of a person is a noun derived from Latin "persona." This signified the mask that actors wore in ancient times that would help to develop the role played by the actor, hence *persona dramatis*. The word then evolved and became synonymous with personality with the idea of individuality and then subsequently the individual. Each individual has a unique face and features which extend down to the submolecular and genetic level. In cultures and races there is a tremendous diversity of facial features that make each one unique yet consistent with that race, each with their own definition of attractiveness and beauty. Plastic surgery not only now restores but also enhances people's features to maintain attractiveness and beauty.

There is also a large functional component to plastic surgery. This has been expanded to all parts of the body and particularly the hands, which are so fundamental to our daily activities. Now the term plastic surgery goes beyond the mere acts of surgery but extends now to the ability to not only mold flesh but grow, stretch and engineer tissue to replace those of missing elements.

The aesthetic appearance of the face is based not only on the harmonious proportions of the eyes, nose and mouth, but also on their relationship to the underlying bony skeleton of the mandible, maxilla, and cranium. Reconstructive surgery and aesthetic surgery run a common course, and in many ways the two are indistinguishable. Reconstruction techniques used to only correct the deformed or abnormal also can improve aesthetic proportion. The expectations of patients with severe deformities are similar to those requesting aesthetic procedures. Despite the limitations of surgery, patients often desire not merely to have a normal appearance, but to be beautiful.

Ideal results in aesthetic plastic surgery are based partly on scientific, partly on artistic solutions. Scientifically, the plastic surgeon relies on numerous standards, cephalometric tracings, and measurements to achieve normal or aesthetic results. The scientific numbers, however, cannot realize a beautiful result; they serve only as guidelines. The aesthetic success of a procedure depends on highlighting the unique proportions or characteristics of the face to reflect its individual character and beauty.

Since Greco-Roman times, artists have used rules of simple proportions, or canons, to describe the ideal human figure. One of the most frequently cited in medical literature is derived from Pythagorean mathematics describing a ration of 1:1, 618, often called the "golden section." This relationship constant, called phi in recognition of the Greek sculptor, Phidias, was derived by means of a ruler and a compass. The orderly mathematic progression of these numbers make triangles, spirals, and arcs, the proportions of which are found in the natural world in sea shells, flower shapes, and other forms, even the spiral growth pattern of the human mandible. The unique mathematic progression of these numbers results in a pattern of "beautiful" relationships that can be applied to the analysis and reconstruction of the human face. The height and width of the face, canthi of the eyes, alar rim of the nose, width of the mouth, height of the lips, and angle of the chin are among the elements whose individual proportions and interrelationships contribute to aesthetic appearance.

Leonardo da Vinci, both artist and scientist, carefully delineated the degree of variation in "ideal" human morphologic forms. His work and that of other artists helped refine proportional canons. Although these canons were developed and used by artists, there was scientific need for this information and so the study of anthropometry, the measurement of living subjects, evolved. Anthropometry came into general use in the past century and provided a quantitative tool for describing the human body and, in particular, the human face. Indices were created to metrically describe the shape, contour, and proportions of the human face in a less subjective manner. This allowed anatomists and anthropologists to determine average or "ideals" for various populations, races, and ethnic groups.

Modern technology allows surgeons to restore form and function creating those contours and shapes that artists deem normal or even attractive. Today plastic surgery includes using small devices known as bone distractors to stretch bones and grow bones. Distractors often have the side effect of also enlarging some of the surrounding tissue, such as muscle and skin, and stretching nerves. Implanting this simple device lets us do things we can't do with standard types of surgery. We actually program tissue to change with these devices.

We are also working in laboratories to actually create new tissue from stem cells. We use tissue to create bone or cartilage when it is needed. We are also using other technologies to replace missing parts or parts that have been lost because of cancer or trauma.

Ultimately, plastic surgery, like all other surgery, will be done through injection of cells, modification of genes, and other advances.

While people usually associate plastic surgery with anti-aging measures, that will eventually be accomplished by manipulating hormones, tissue, and the actual genes that cause us to age. They'll be modified so people can live longer, and their quality of life will be better.

Plastic Surgery Subspecialties

Plastic surgery is a very diverse specialty. Within the specialty itself, we have people who deal only with aesthetic reconstruction of the face or restoration of the face. We have people who do only breast surgery – to enlarge or reduce the breasts or reconstruct them after cancer. Other plastic surgeons deal with congenital anomalies such as cleft lip and palate or more extensive craniofacial anomalies and vascular malformations. We have people who do body contouring, which reshapes arms, legs, and the abdomen.

There is a new branch of surgery that treats formerly obese people. That surgery is now very common. People are losing large amounts of weight, and they then need to deal with the issues of all the extra soft tissue and the distortions and deformities that result from losing massive tissue volume as well as developing deformities from the laxity of the overall skin structures. This results in the need for reshaping and recontouring to have a much more aesthetically balanced shape that includes the trunk, arms and legs.

There are surgeons who do only hand surgery, resolving congenital and traumatic hand problems. This subspecialty is actually a significant area of practice in plastic surgery: People who have injured their extremities account for about 40 percent of emergency room visits. With microscopic techniques the ability to replant fingers and limbs have now become commonplace at most trauma centers.

Surgeons who deal with cleft lip and palate and craniofacial anomalies do reconstruction of the skull and the jaw. When the neurocranium is involved, oftentimes the neurosurgeon is assisting the craniofacial surgeon to carry out the complete reconstruction. This surgery often involves the association with a neurosurgeon to carry out the complete reconstruction. Oral surgeons and maxillofacial surgeons also assist in the reconstruction of the mid-face, lower face and mandible.

Microsurgeons are those who use the techniques of moving large blocks of tissue – many times composed of skin, muscle and bone – to different areas for reconstruction of massive tissue loss or cancer reconstruction. Using the microscope over the operative site, they can reconnect the blood vessels and nerves from the new blocks of tissue to restore the parts, volume and form of the missing area.

The Captain of the Ship

The role of a surgeon is similar to that of the captain of a ship. He creates the design, devises the treatment plan, and guides the execution. Many of the things I do involve multidisciplinary types of specialties. For example, if my patient is a child with a congenital cleft lip and palate deformity, we actually compose a team that will involve pediatric ear, nose, and throat doctors, speech therapists, geneticists, oral surgeons, dentists, and audiologists, just to mention a few specialties.

We take that child from infancy to adulthood, offering help in dealing with the variety of issues that confront him or her. The surgeon is actually the team captain, or director, who helps guide where the child should go next in the treatment plan. Sometimes the plastic surgeon is more involved in the beginning and the end of the facial restoration, and others help by working on the functional aspects, such as hearing; they might place tubes in the child's ears or evaluate the hearing with audiology examinations.

Usually the surgeon decides how he would like his team composed and how he would like his team to be formed. Different teams have different philosophies, often reflecting the director's, or surgeon's, point of view. I base my decisions on the talent and expertise I have around me and try to pick the best I can to achieve synergy, where the results of our combined efforts as a team are better than we could have achieved as a number of individuals working separately.

Qualities of a Successful Plastic Surgeon

Most plastic surgeons have a very artistic bent in their whole perception of life. They look at form and function. When most surgeons operate, the patient can't see the end result of their work, although they can often appreciate it functionally. But most of the work of plastic surgeons is very visible – often the face you are looking at.

As a plastic surgeon, you must have the ability to resolve whatever problem you are dealing with to a level of quality that is esthetically acceptable to the patient. Most patients with an injury or a birth defect want to look the best they possibly can. There is a certain demand for quality in the artistic rendering of the face you are dealing with. Another layer deals with the function, which has to be appropriate, as well.

A plastic surgeon has to have a solid grasp of the history and evolution of plastic surgery. If we are presented with a very challenging problem, we will go back to see what other giants in the field have done to try to resolve a similar problem.

Today we are faced with problems that are increasingly challenging because of advances in other areas of medicine. For example, people survive car crashes and airplane crashes in better conditions than they did in the past, not only because of improved safety standards of equipment and vehicles, but also because of improvements in medicine. We now have the technology, skills, and expertise to help some people with birth defects survive beyond the early infant years to a point where they can be comfortable in society.

Sometimes we are faced with a challenge no one else has ever seen. Then we have to use our imagination and our background and our expertise to come up with a viable treatment plan that will work to restore that person's life.

If we reach a point where we can devise accurate, reproducible treatment plans for patients, ultimately giving them pleasing, satisfactory results, then we are successful. The goal is to reproduce your technology and techniques satisfactorily on the majority of patients. Everything in medicine is a bell curve, but if you can shift that curve so that your success rate continuously and consistently improves, producing satisfactory outcomes with minimal problems or morbidity, then you are successful.

We also must keep in mind that we can't become so absorbed in our field that we lose sight of family and friends. Everything in life is a balance – a truth that many of us tend to forget because of the long hours we have to work to accomplish what we feel we need to do. For me, balancing the personal and the professional parts of life is very difficult. I have a great interest in teaching, and I also get deeply involved with the administration process of medicine, so my interest is not all clinical.

I wish I could do a better job of balancing. In a world that becomes more complex, you think you have all the new technology to make your life easier – but I find I have less time now than I did before we had all these new technologies. Our operating times have shortened, and the whole process is carried out in a much better, safer, and more efficient fashion. As humans, however, we tend to do more work when we have more time.

Managing Expectations through Open Communication

Whether the surgery is esthetic or reconstructive, you have to develop a path for communication with your patient and a rapport that is as comfortable as possible. Most patients today are very intelligent. They surf the Internet and are aware of what is available. Often they will have done research and networked with organizations or other individuals who have problems or issues similar to theirs or experience in dealing with similar issues.

I need to know what the patient actually knows about their particular issue or problem, whether it is a facelift or a complex facial problem. Educating the patient on their needs and the resolution of their issues is very important. You have to make sure their expectations are realistic.

Often women in their 80s bring a picture of themselves taken when they were 18 or 20 and say they want to look like that again. The process of aging is global; that is, it affects every cell in our bodies. Some of the effects are unchangeable or irreversible, although I can redo some of the stigmata associated with aging, and I tell the patient how we can accomplish that. Whether the solution is simple or complex, you have to be able to understand what the patient is asking, and the patient has to be able to understand what you tell them.

If a patient has any doubts about a procedure, sometimes we will have them talk with other individuals or other doctors for a second or third opinion so they can get a better understanding and perhaps find someone with whom they have a better rapport. I often will give patients literature, material I have written, or other people have written, to help them understand the whole process. I try to educate the patient; once they are educated, it is much easier for me to communicate with them.

Process of Treating a Patient

Essentially a patient calls the office for an appointment, and they are usually asked what particular issues they want evaluated or discussed. At their appointment, we evaluate the patient, take a history, and do a physical examination.

Then the education process starts. I give the patient options and treatment plans that are available to them because I like to give patients choices. I then try to get a feel for where they want to go with the procedure. I will give them literature and sometimes show them pictures from my clinical books or some of the textbooks I have written to try to give them further information.

I often tell patients to go home and think about what they want to do and what we've covered because they often hear or remember only about 40 percent of what you tell them in that first visit. If it is appropriate, we will bring them back to re-discuss and re-evaluate the options. By that time the patients have a better understanding of the whole picture, and if it is appropriate, we will then proceed with surgery.

As you're talking with and listening to your patient, if you realize they actually need a psychiatrist instead of a plastic surgeon, you should recognize this need and refer them to a psychiatrist. You have to be a doctor. Some people come to a plastic surgeon for a quick fix, but that may not be appropriate for them. You need to be able to be a good doctor first, and a good listener, and try to help the patient in the most appropriate way. It all goes back to the Hippocratic Oath, though many of us sometimes tend to forget that.

When a patient presents us with a problem we have never experienced before, sometimes we share that person's condition with others in the field whom you respect for their opinions. Many doctors and colleagues are very willing to share their expertise and advice. Sometimes the result is a unique solution you had not thought of before.

Helping Patients Deal with Risks

There are the usual medical risks associated with surgery, which include anesthetic problems and allergic reactions. If the surgery is very complex, there could be problems of bleeding or infection, which are usually low, but depending on the complexity of the issues, you may have people who are at a higher risk than others.

Beyond those risks, you have the healing process to get through. Most people feel that when the operation is over, they are finished. But the healing process goes on from weeks to months. It may take that long for the patient to see the final results.

There is often a psychological curve that moves along with the healing process. Many patients have a slight degree of depression right after surgery because when they look in the mirror, they are bruised black and blue and swollen, and they don't recognize themselves. But once they see the bruising go away and the swelling go down, their features start to return, and they get very excited. The process continues, and as they improve, they actually become happy and pleased.

We help patients manage all of the phases, from pre-surgery through surgery and healing. Each phase is important; each is associated with its own needs and unique features. You must help the patient through each of these phases to end up with a happy patient.

Plastic surgeons have learned through their training how to minimize and hide incisions. Technology has further assisted by allowing us to use instruments that require only small incisions so we can work under the skin and avoid making numerous incisions. We also use products on incisions to make them heal better with less scarring.

I tend to pre-treat patients with certain homeopathic agents that we know reduce swelling and bruising, as well as other agents that enhance wound healing. Using this method, we pre-treat patients so that their bodies are induced to accelerate healing even before surgery takes place.

During surgery we use different medications, again to reduce bruising and swelling and speed up the healing process as much as possible.

During the postoperative period, we use other technologies. We are even looking into infrared technology, which the Defense Department is evaluating to try to treat soldiers who are injured on the field. We can apply the military technology to everyday surgery.

We are always looking at new ways of controlling physiology and the body's ability to recover from surgery.

When Scarring Becomes an Issue

Once the scar is mature, it is stable. The problem is that some people have certain genetic compositions that cause the scar to take on a much nastier appearance. They don't have the elements that will actually allow the cells that produce the scar to shut off; the result is that they lay down scar on top of scar and collagen on top of collagen. This process causes a tremendous deformity that is a problem symptomatically.

This problem often happens in burn patients whose burns have altered permanently the state of the burned skin. I have taken care of pilots who fought in the Battle of London in World War II who continued to suffer from the long-term effects of their scars, which were constantly contracting and altering even though the scars were mature. The dynamic nature of scars is another field that people are constantly researching. Although we are developing a better understanding of it, we don't quite have the ability to control it as effectively as we would like to.

Keeping Up-to-Date with Technology

Meetings and relevant literature help us keep up with all of the new technological developments. Often we have people from the medical technology companies come in to demonstrate the advances their companies have made and how to use them.

At the meetings, some of the scientific papers that are presented will also have technical support in the exhibit area, where you can talk about the new technology with the manufacturers or the technicians to get a clearer understanding of how it works and what it can do. Many companies will send a representative to you to help with your specific needs. There are many ways to keep up with the technology, and obviously it's critical that we learn to use the new technologies that represent advances and improvements.

As far as surgical techniques are concerned, we are still in the Middle Ages in that we still have to make incisions, and we have to make the incisions heal afterward. Although we are much better at controlling those processes, we still are trying to understand their basic molecular biology. Once we get a better handle on that, we can control it better.

We all learn from each other. The individuals who impress me most are those who have stood on the shoulders of giants, learned from them, and carried their knowledge to a higher level. I truly admire doctors who are less egotistical, who are part of a science and a profession that allow us to share our knowledge among the entire group so we can all benefit from that knowledge – to the ultimate benefit of our patients.

The best piece of advice with respect to practicing plastic surgery is to keep your mind open and keep learning. Plastic surgery is a dynamic process. Many things I have learned in the past 20 years are obsolete or have changed dramatically or philosophically or have totally reorganized. You must keep learning.

From Good to Great

People should train well to do what they are expected to do or what they have aspired to do. When you take shortcuts, you can shortchange both the patients and yourself. Many times that will reflect badly on the whole field of plastic surgery, or even medicine in general. Usually when you take a shortcut, it fails to achieve what you wanted it to do.

As with many endeavors, you need an innate ability that allows you to be a successful plastic surgeon. Different facets require different talents, but most plastic surgeons are artistic either in their ability to perceive and think in three-dimensional shapes and forms, or in basing their esthetic canons on the same artistic canons that artists and sculptors such as Michelangelo used to create human forms and define beauty.

Physical beauty is elusive, but it can be reduced to some simple mathematical formulas that have been around for thousands of years. Plastic surgeons tend to embrace those ideals. Many of us are artists in different media. We have a strong artistic interest to begin with, but not all are good painters or sculptors. Understanding at least what an artist looks at and, of course, understanding the execution to achieve that ideal is crucial – this understanding is what makes plastic surgery. In the Middle Ages in order for the great artists and sculptors of the time to more accurately represent the human body, the artists themselves would take human anatomy dissections in order to replicate the proper shape and form that is the science to create the ultimate accurate form and shape.

Beyond that minimum understanding, which any good plastic surgeon can achieve, a great plastic surgeon can perform plastic surgery with results that are far superior esthetically and functionally than anyone else.

Changes in Plastic Surgery

Technology and culture have driven changes in plastic surgery. Technology has allowed us to do things more easily and safely, and with more minimally invasive techniques to accomplish results that otherwise would have required major operations. Liposuction, for example, which requires small incisions, is a very safe application of aspirating fat cells and re-contouring the body.

Before liposuction, surgeons had to make circumferential incisions around the body, the legs, and the arms, leading to a much bloodier, more dangerous operation with horrendous scarring and a highly inferior result. We have taken something that was very complex to something that is easy and safe, with a fast recovery and more predictable, favorable results.

In the next five years, there will be a greater emphasis on the total body. People spend a great deal of money to look younger, but their issues are actually more global than they usually like to admit – they also need to change their lifestyle, nutrition, and probably many habits. Just staying out of the sun, for instance, will do much to prevent aging.

Educating the public on what makes a more healthful lifestyle is key. People are much more interested in changing their lifestyle and looking better and fitter and improving their quality of life.

Also, a growing field of medicine, of which plastic surgeons are usually a part, is the field of anti-aging medicine. People truly want to prolong their lives and maintain a high quality of life for as long as possible. That involves manipulation of some of the natural hormones and elements in our bodies that age depletes.

In other specialties, surgeons are using robots, which require very small incisions and are guided by the use of machines that allow minimally invasive surgery. The result is less trauma to surrounding tissues and a much faster recovery.

The goal of surgery is for it to evolve into a non-surgical specialty. Already people can swallow capsules that have cameras inside that photograph the entire digestive system as it moves through. Robots can do heart surgery with very small incisions, and patients don't even have to go on cardiac bypass. The technology is rapidly evolving into advances of which we never dreamed.

Dr. Dufresne's expertise and interest in aesthetic and reconstructive Plastic Surgery includes cosmetic surgery, cancer and congenital reconstruction and has won him critical acclaim and several awards. In addition to recognition of his clinical and research work, he has been cited in regional and national magazines as among the best Doctors in Washington since 1986, along with being cited in Who's Who in Medical Specialties, Who's Who in Medicine and Healthcare, and Best Doctors in America.

He has lectured nationally and internationally and written his own textbook on plastic surgery. He has also published extensively in journals and other textbooks in the field.

Dr. Dufresne has been a past Assistant Professor in Neurosurgery at The Johns Hopkins University and Medical Institutions, Director of the Facial Rehabilitation Center at the Children's Hospital and The

Johns Hopkins Hospital in Baltimore and the Ear Deformity Clinic for The Johns Hopkins Hospital. Dr. Dufresne has also been the Chief of Plastic Surgery Service at the Loch Raven VA Medical Center and attending consultant at the University of Maryland and Maryland Institute of Emergency Medical Services (MIEMS – Shock Trauma Center of Baltimore).

Dedication *- Dedicated to my professors, patients' families and especially to my patients themselves who helped to inspire us each day. They have also taught us a great deal, each in his own way. I hope to carry on my patients' thoughts, ideas and dreams in order to help future patients.*

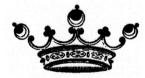

The Rewards of Plastic Surgery

Barry J. Cohen, M.D., FACS

Board Certified Plastic Surgeon
Suburban, Sibley, Montgomery General,
Shady Grove, and Holy Cross Hospitals &
The Washington Hospital Center

The Science of Aesthetic Medicine – The Artistry of Change

It has long been said that beauty is in the eye of the beholder. Surely the most important beholder is you. Whether you accept it or not, we live in a society where looks count. How you feel about the way you look sends off a signal to the world that you are confident, successful, and content in your own skin. In aesthetic plastic surgery, the most rewarding outcome I can achieve is a happy and satisfied patient.

The art of being a good aesthetic plastic surgeon has as much to do with having an eye for what things can and should be done to people physically as it does with taking care of the psyche of each patient as an individual. Everyone has unique needs, both physical and emotional. In many ways, we can be considered psychiatrists with scalpels. I do not mean to imply that most cosmetic surgery patients are mentally ill, but people have different motivations for aesthetic improvement. Some reasons for having cosmetic procedures are well founded, and some are clearly not. Figuring out the motivations of people is as much an art as the surgery itself. The role of the aesthetic plastic surgeon is not only to decide what things can be done that will improve the patient's appearance, but equally as important is defining what things should be done and what things should not be done. The fact that we have mastered a technique, and the patient standing before us is a candidate for that procedure, does not mandate that it is the right operation for that patient. Above all, communication is the key to a successful and rewarding doctor-patient relationship.

Surgery is not a perfect science. Yet, the science of plastic surgery is critical at several levels. As a surgeon, you have to be technically competent and have mastered tried and true surgical methods and know your anatomy. Without these basic skills, everything else won't matter. You have to be able to know instinctively what should be accomplished aesthetically, and have the practical skills to manage it.

Therein lies the major difference between plastic surgery and other surgical specialties. We are trained to look at the face and body in functional terms as well as aesthetic terms. For the most part, plastic surgeons are not saving lives. We are not removing life threatening tumors or performing miracles with open heart surgery. We are, however, entrusted with improving the quality of life of our patients. Aside from the obvious area of cosmetic surgery, we are trained to improve congenital deformities like cleft lips and in breast reconstruction.

Technologically Speaking

To remain current on technological advances, I read constantly, as any physician must. I read a handful of journals every month that are relevant to my practice, and I regularly attend meetings and conferences, which is how most of us keep up with this ever changing specialty. I talk to my colleagues across the country to learn about what other people are doing. Staying current with the medical literature and following clinical studies allows me to offer my patients the most effective state-of-the-art techniques and technologies, which are constantly upgraded. My rule is never to be the first or the last surgeon using any particular product or procedure. I prefer to adapt established techniques that are safe and effective for my patients, and the artistry entails adding your personal signature or twist to a method to bring it up a notch.

Fortunately, modern advances in cosmetic surgery have made it possible to enhance your appearance safely, effectively, with less pain, bruising and shorter recovery times. Another arena that offers new challenges in this field is the science of wound healing and scar reduction. As plastic surgeons we are always interested in finding better ways to manage scars and improve the healing process for our patients.

Lasers and light sources are perhaps the biggest buzzwords in aesthetic medicine today. These systems are being used to treat a growing number of conditions including hair removal, spider veins and brown spots or age spots on the face, chest, and hands and legs, as well as active acne, acne scarring and improvements in skin texture and discoloration. There are many systems on the market that work well, and produce satisfactory results, but usually only after a series of multiple treatments.

In plastic surgery, lasers are predominantly used for skin resurfacing. The carbon dioxide or CO2 laser, which is the gold standard for that treatment, leaves patients very red, and there is a real risk of having permanent de-pigmentation. Although there have been many alternative technologies that have come to market, the only one that truly stands out is the CO2 laser. However, deeper lasers come with greater risks and longer downtime, and patients simply are not willing to accept this. I am looking forward to better laser technology for skin resurfacing. None of the technologies on the market is fabulous, and many lasers do not produce very dramatic results. Real improvements in laser technology will continue to be developed and this is an area that will offer significant advancements for our field. I always advise my patients not to get too concerned with attempting to navigate the differences and nuances of laser technologies. Many physicians don't even understand the physics themselves. The technology changes far too quickly for the average lay person to keep up. The best advice is to find a good laser surgeon and follow his recommendations for your individual concerns and skin type.

The flipside of the growth in aesthetic surgery is the movement away from reconstructive surgery. I consider this to be an unfortunate development because of the accompanying loss of reconstructive skills. As plastic surgeons, we have spent many years undergoing extensive training to do hand surgery, facial reconstruction, burn reconstruction, microsurgery, and breast reconstruction. Many of my colleagues are giving up doing those procedures completely. This change has had a tremendous negative impact on plastic surgery. Reconstructive surgery has become something that is done mostly by faculty in university hospitals, and it will be less available in the real world – in community hospitals, where it has routinely been done. It limits people's options for where they can go to get that kind of surgery. I believe that the pendulum will ultimately swing back, but regrettably not before we have lost many skilled surgeons from the specialty of plastic surgery

Current Trends and New Developments

A common misconception of cosmetic surgery is that once you have a facelift, you'll have to keep having them. In fact, the opposite is true. If you ask how long a facelift will last, the answer is forever. You will always look better for having had a lift at whatever stage you do it. As the face continually changes with age, the benefits of having undergone surgery will ensure that you will look younger than your chronological age. Cosmetic surgery of the face involves far more than just the basic garden variety facelift today.

There are many non-surgical minimally invasive rejuvenative procedures that have revolutionized the field of aesthetic plastic surgery in recent years. The real growth in the field is being driven by scientific advancements and new technologies, as well as consumer demands for less invasive procedures with shorter healing times.

Botulinum toxin, popularly known as BOTOX® for example, was approved by the FDA in 2002 for cosmetic uses. Botulinum toxin has the distinction of being the only injectable that is preventative as well as corrective. Just one treatment brings a noticeable improvement in the softening of facial lines. Botulinum toxin has become the foundation of an early battle against visible aging. Unlike fillers that temporarily plump up creases but don't really prevent them from getting deeper or stop new ones from forming, it slows down the formation of new facial lines. Combining Botulinum toxin to stop new lines from forming, with treatments for the creases that are already there, is the best comprehensive approach to forestall surgery. The toxin acts on the junctions between nerves and muscles, preventing the release of a chemical messenger called acetylcholine from the nerve endings. Tiny amounts are injected into a specific facial muscle so only the targeted impulse of that muscle will be blocked, causing a local relaxation. It acts as a muscle blockade to immobilize the underlying cause of the unwanted lines – muscle contractions – and prevent 'wrinkly' expressions. Since it can no longer make the offending facial expression, the lines gradually smooth out from disuse and new creases will form at a slower rate. Other muscles that are not treated are not affected to maintain a natural look and expressions. It may not be as effective on lines that are not entirely caused by the action of a muscle, i.e. the nasal labial folds that are formed by a combination of muscle action and the weight of sagging skin. Some areas are less effective because the muscles are needed for expression and important functions like eating, kissing, and opening the eyes. The goal is not to knock out every muscle twinge; but rather an overall softening of dynamic facial lines that looks natural and refreshed.

The dermal filler market has been expanding rapidly around the world, and in November 2003, the FDA panel is expected to rule on several new filling substances. Wrinkle fillers turn up on the market constantly, but it takes time to establish the long-term safety of newly released formulas. The approval of these substances varies from country to country. New fillers are under clinical investigation all the time, and products with a high incidence of reactions and complications have difficulty getting approval in America.

In the US, they are considered medical devices and fall under the domain of the FDA, which has more stringent requirements than its European or Canadian counterparts. I am always very cautious about introducing a new wrinkle filler treatment into my practice, unless the safety data has been well established. I advise my patients to wait until it has been used safely for three to five years before having it injected into your face. The newest product may not always be the best available and doctors need time to determine the advantages and/or disadvantages of any new product in comparison to existing fillers on the market. The results may look fine right now, but you'll want to know that as you age and your skin thins, you won't see or feel lumps and bumps hardening due to the use of synthetic particles. Generally, the longer lasting filling substances are, the more complications are possible. The safest wrinkle filler treatments are generally those that have the longest and best track record, meaning more people have had treatments successfully.

Selecting a Qualified Aesthetic Plastic Surgeon

There is much consumer confusion today about the various medical specialties and the credentialing process for doctors performing cosmetic procedures. More and more practitioners are moving to aesthetic medicine from general surgery and family practice because insurance companies have reduced the rates they pay for medical care today. Due to the influence of managed care on the practice of medicine, it has become increasingly difficult for doctors and surgeons to make a living and to avoid the syndrome of the dreaded $15 co-pay. Therefore, the aesthetic arena has become more attractive and more competitive.

Finding a doctor who is board-certified by an American Board of Medical Specialties (www.abms.org) accredited board in his particular specialty is an excellent place to start. Board certification in plastic surgery is difficult to obtain and maintain. It is considered one of the most grueling board-certification processes of all the specialties. Board certification should never be considered a guarantee of excellence, but rather a minimum requirement that assures some degree of clinical excellence. The other important component is aesthetics. Just because a plastic surgeon is board certified does not mean he is very good or experienced at aesthetic surgery.

Consumers can also check with their State Medical Boards which maintain open repositories of complaints against doctors, as well as listings of doctors who have had malpractice claims filed against them. Evidence of one isolated lawsuit should not necessarily be a reason to eliminate any doctor from your list. We live in a litigious society where people bring lawsuits for no valid reason at all, so it should come as no surprise that patients sue doctors every day for many reasons that are not malpractice.

If you have been considering having cosmetic surgery, you have probably been collecting names of doctors from friends, other physicians, hairstylists, along with clippings from magazines and newspapers, and every source has its own favorites. In the D.C. area, The Washingtonian magazine runs a list of the top doctors every couple of years in which physicians nominate their peers based on whom they would send their family members to. Although recommendations from friends and acquaintances can be helpful, it isn't fair to judge a doctor on the basis of one isolated recommendation or condemnation either. The most important credential a doctor has is his professional reputation.

Once you get past the basics in terms of credentials, a person considering plastic surgery needs to find a practitioner with whom he or she connects on an emotional or personal level. It's more than just finding someone who does good work; there are many doctors and surgeons who fit that bill. It is a matter of being able to click with the doctor and feel confident that he understands what you want and can deliver it.

Personality Matters

Historically, people tend to think of surgeons as falling short in the category of bedside manner. Many of my colleagues fall into two types. The paternalistic plastic surgeons tell each patient to put himself into their brilliant, talented, artistic hands, and they will transform her into whatever his vision of her happens to be. Then there are doctors like me, who communicate with the patient and come up with a treatment plan based on what the patient wants, with some guidance from the surgeon as to what is possible to achieve and how to get there. Ideally, my role as a plastic surgeon is as a team member with the patient and the nurse and anyone else involved; i.e. a spouse or significant other. Ultimately, the primary goal is to achieve the appearance the patient wants. I am only the facilitator.

I personally believe the role of the surgeon is to be a partner with the patient. Certain qualities in a plastic surgeon's personality predispose him or her to success with patients. A good sense of humor, a lack of arrogance, and empathy for patients' concerns are all high on the list. I believe a doctor who does not take himself or herself overly seriously but who, at the same time, takes patients' concerns very seriously, Even issues that are seemingly insignificant is paramount in the mind of the patient. Surgeons need to keep their mind as well as their ears open to dealing with patient fears and concerns. The most minor procedure takes on major importance to the person undergoing it, and to his or her family and loved ones.

It is very easy for doctors, who see things over and over again, to minimize a complaint or dismiss a patient's question as trivial. This attitude inevitably leads to patient dissatisfaction. Giving a patient your undivided attention and making her feel that she is the only person in your universe at that moment is critical. As cosmetic surgeons, we are expected to give patients the "warm and fuzzies," which is a colloquial term, but it fits. We are in a service industry; cosmetic procedures are elective and considered a luxury purchase. Patients have many choices today, and they can go anywhere.

For doctors entering the specialty of aesthetic medicine, working with good plastic surgeons who are great teachers is the best way to learn what makes the difference between an average practitioner and an outstanding one. The place to learn the nuances of aesthetic plastic surgery is in day to day practice in the real world, not during your residency. When I started out on my own, I learned things predominantly the hard way. As an established surgeon now, I am blessed with the opportunity to work with junior colleagues and offer them the benefit of my experience. My younger associates have had the advantage of learning from my mistakes; technically in surgery, as well as in how to run a practice, internal and external marketing, staffing, training, and patient selection. I think they would all agree that I have forged many passages.

From Initial Consultation to the Post-Op Phase

My practice is predominantly cosmetic surgery and, unlike the practice of a general surgeon or an internist, the diagnosis, for the most part, is patient-driven. People who come in for an initial consultation usually have a specific complaint; for example, their breasts are too small, or their eyes are sagging, or they dislike their droopy neck, or they have too much fat on their hips. When a new patient arrives, I introduce myself to them informally using my first name: "Hi, I'm Barry." I ask what is bothering them, and they tell me. For example, if their chief complaint is that their breasts are too small, treatment would most likely be limited to breast implants.

The next step is to explain the procedure in detail and review the options in terms of anesthesia, surgical facility, technique or method, scar pattern and results. You need to know the basics of the procedure and how they apply directly to you specifically. Understanding the limitations of the procedure is also crucial. Skin type, degree of skin elasticity, individual healing, bone structure, general health, dental health, previous surgery to the area, and many other factors will determine to some extent the quality of the result you can expect.

After they have learned about what the surgery entails, I take them through the litany of risks and complications. It is essential not to sugarcoat procedures for patients. It is always better to under promise for expectations and over-deliver on results. I also cover the alternatives for every surgical procedure. Today, there is more than one way to rejuvenate the eyelids, for example. There are several surgical techniques that may be appropriate, plus a handful of non-invasive treatments including botulinum toxin, fillers, lasers and chemical peels that may accomplish the patient's goals. It is the surgeon's responsibility to review most if not all of these. There are times when the patient may not be ready emotionally or cannot afford to take the time to have surgery at this stage. We can often suggest non-surgical alternatives that may address at least some of their immediate concerns. For instance, for fat reduction of the torso, there is liposuction, a mini-tummy tuck or a full tummy tuck. I routinely explain all of these procedures, how they differ in terms of recovery, outcome and cost factors. After carefully reviewing the advantages and disadvantages for each and the downtime involved, I will make my recommendation as to which would be preferable for that particular patient. My job is to describe all the options, but ultimately, the patient has to decide how to proceed.

My staff and I also spend considerable time explaining the post-operative course with patients so they understand what to expect and what the psychological impact may be after specific procedures. I insist that my patients come back again to our office at least once if not more to make sure they have had all their questions answered. We like our patients to be very well prepared before surgery to make the entire process run smoothly for them and for us.

Staying in touch with patients is of paramount importance. I take care to ensure that they never feel isolated or afraid to contact us when they need something. I am one of a rare breed of plastic surgeons who are very computer literate and carry my Blackberry with me at all times. My business card has my email address on it, and I often answer email at 11 o'clock at night. Email is a great communication channel for patients because they don't have to feel that they are bothering me, and I can get back to them quickly. Post-operatively, I call my patients on the night of surgery to see how they are doing and reassure them. The days are usually very busy, so having extensions of me – that is, highly trained nurses who are extremely familiar with the surgery and my protocols – is very helpful. Many of them have had the procedure themselves, and they are very effective in answering questions for patients and handling their needs.

Discussing Risks & Complications

It is every patient's right to be informed of the potential risks and complications of any medical procedure. Your doctor should make every effort to minimize complications; however, it is not possible to eliminate the potential for all negative effects from occurring. With any medical or surgical procedure, there is always a possibility of unexpected or unwanted events. No absolute guarantees as to the final result can ever be given by any physician. The ultimate decision to proceed rests with the patient, after the doctor has made a conscientious effort to explain every aspect of the procedure to the patient. Your doctor has a legal and ethical responsibility to explain these potential complications in detail so that you are well informed about what could go wrong and what to watch out for.

There are specific risks ascribed to each procedure, but infection, bleeding, and scarring are the most common across the board in plastic surgery. The risks of cosmetic surgery can be divided into two main groups: those that are common after all operations, and those that are unique to a specific technique or procedure. It is also important to factor in the variables of your individual health status, your age, skin quality, gender, and your medical history. Clearly a younger patient in prime health will have less risk than an older patient with a history of high blood pressure. Males are more prone to bleeding because they have a rich blood supply and thicker skin. Thin skinned patients may be more prone to bruising. The most common risks of cosmetic procedures include swelling, bruising, bleeding, infection, prolonged numbness, and a reaction to anesthesia. General surgical complications may include hematoma, which is a blood clot; seroma, which is a collection of clear fluid; nerve damage, scar tissue formation, asymmetries, and irregularities. Infections are rare and are typically treated with a course of antibiotics. It is common to be prescribed an antibiotic before and/or after surgery to guard against infection.

If you are having a surgery that involves placing an implant or graft, there is always the possibility of extrusion, whereby the implant works its way up to the surface of the skin, and capsular contracture, which is an excess tightening of scar tissue that forms around the implant. Breast implants have their own set of risks. Liposuction has a different set of risks. Other common risks include asymmetry or irregularities and these can apply to all procedures. According to national statistics, the need for revisions after liposuction is about one in three. I tell my patients preoperatively that there is a slight possibility that a revision will be required or requested, and with liposuction, it would be performed about six months after surgery. For other procedures, like eyelids or facelifts, it will vary from three months to one year in some cases. Revisions are rare, and I normally don't charge the patients to do a minor touch-up like a scar revision in the office under local anesthesia. If they need to go back into the surgicenter under anesthesia, then there is a nominal facility and anesthesiologist's fee incurred.

Unfortunately, every plastic surgeon has some patients who are not happy with the results, and each for a different reason. Sometimes the surgery has a less than ideal outcome resulting from postoperative infection, bleeding or poor skin tone. It can happen even to the most skilled surgeon, although every effort should be made to minimize the incidence of unforeseen problems both pre and post-op as well as during the actual surgery. The patient selection process can be a complicated one. Even after I have explained what the proposed surgery can and cannot accomplish, some patients still may harbor extremely unrealistic expectations. These patients will not be happy with the results of cosmetic surgery and would be better off postponing or opting not to have it done at all. Although patients sign consent forms that stipulate the risks and complications of their proposed surgery, it is human nature to believe those risks and complications happen only to other patients, never to you. Being totally honest and forthcoming with patients is of paramount importance. I have always found that patients respect you for it and will trust you more because of your candor. They are also not always expecting it from a surgeon, so in can be a welcome surprise.

Plastic surgeons do not have a magic wand they can wave at will. There are no miracles to be had. The most widespread misconception is that plastic surgery is scarless. Any time you make an incision, it leaves a scar and complications can occur. People come in thinking a plastic surgeon can get rid of a scar they have or perform some surgery without producing a scar, but that simply cannot happen. It takes from three to six months to get over most surgeries, before swelling disappears and scars mature. It is not uncommon for scars to take a year to mature. That is the most difficult point to get across. Some patients expect immediate gratification, and it just is not possible.

Many factors other than technique and talent are involved in surgical outcomes, many of which are beyond any doctor's control. We are only human.

Separating the Good from the Great

Several qualities make a great surgeon. Consistency in outcome is number one, and that comes from doing many surgeries. There is no substitute for experience. Great surgeons are able to critique their own work and improve their performance based on both positive and negative outcomes. Throughout history, some of the great plastic surgeons have had humility and the ability to connect with all patients on their own level. The patient may be a college professor, an attorney or a blue-collar worker. An experienced surgeon needs to be able to change his approach to suit individuals based on their needs, not solely his own.

Another important quality is to be open to adopting new techniques and improving your existing methods, while at the same time, not necessarily being the first surgeon to jump on the bandwagon without a healthy degree of caution. I can give you a host of examples in which a surgeon has seen something new that is published and immediately jumps to sell the procedure, but the results are not necessarily better or even as good as previous techniques. There are instances when surgeons publish their newest techniques and are then forced to continually change the procedure too much based on a high complication. Unfortunately, the consequences are that many patients may have very unsatisfactory results from techniques that their surgeon learned from attending a course or reading a paper.

As a group, I think we are a very arrogant breed. Many of us are loners who believe we are the best at what we do. Sometimes our egos get in our way. It is rare and refreshing to meet colleagues who are humble enough to say, "That's beyond me," or "I made a mistake," or even admit that other surgeons do nice work also. It also takes a very thick skin to become a leader in this field. You need to put your neck on the line and say and do things others are not willing to say or do. Someone has to execute a procedure, try something new, and be willing to talk about it. Most people are not prepared to do that because it involves taking risks. As a doctor you need to take calculated and informed risks every day. Every time you pick up a scalpel, you are taking a risk. You need the right personality to do that. I don't think it is something that can be learned. It is a quality that you are either born with or not.

Prescription for Success: A Balanced, Well Rounded Life

Doctors use many different yardsticks for success. For many, the ultimate success comes in the form of a very busy practice that is predominantly based on referrals from happy patients. Some surgeons measure success by what they put in the bank or by how far they have risen or whether they are full professors or associate professors in an academic environment. I have built what is now the largest plastic surgery practice in the nation's capital, yet I have managed to maintain a level of patient care that I can be proud of in all four of my offices. As we have grown, taking on qualified associates has helped handle the additional patient population. I like to be able to spend time with each of my patients, without feeling uncomfortably pressured.

Although it is hard to balance being a doctor with having a personal life, I have a wife and four children at home. The biggest accommodation for me was in giving up most reconstructive surgery. I don't take emergency room calls anymore, and I rarely have patients to visit in the hospital. I am often home by six o'clock at night in time to have dinner with my kids and even help with their homework. I make it a point to rarely work on weekends and try to take a week off every two months to be with my family. All of this makes me a better surgeon and a better human being as well.

Dealing with insurance companies is what I dislike most. They are bureaucratic conglomerates that think they know better than doctors what is best for patients. Like most physicians with a conscience, I resent being told by a person who has no medical expertise what is appropriate for my patient, strictly based on economics. For this reason, I no longer do very much reconstructive surgery. However, I have often been known to do an occasional operation at a reduced fee or pro bono if I come across a patient who needs my help. On some level, I do it as much for myself as I do it for that patient. I feed my soul by doing burn reconstruction, which is my true passion and one of the reasons I became a plastic surgeon. Many of these cases are challenging yet very rewarding at the same time, especially when children are involved.

Future Challenges in Aesthetic Medicine

Patients are exceptionally knowledgeable today. For the most part, they cannot be fooled by marketing hype and cheap salesmanship. I enjoy dealing with educated and well-informed patients. They make my job much easier. The Internet has helped consumers become far better informed about their health care choices than ever before. They often come into a doctor's office armed with facts and lists of questions, and already familiar with the latest procedures, products and techniques. However, there is a lot of misleading and contradictory information out there, especially in chat rooms and on commercial cosmetic surgery websites. Patients should beware that anyone can post anything online without being subjected to scrutiny. The most challenging aspect for the future is managing patient expectations.

Perhaps the greatest test is to try to gauge the patient's psyche and emotional readiness for having surgery and going through the recovery phase, and evaluating their true motivation. The initial consultation may last from 15 to 60 minutes. After one brief meeting, I make a decision along with the patient about proceeding with a surgical procedure. I recognize that I am venturing into a partnership with the patient that may change his or her life in some way. The classic example of misplaced motivation is a person going through a divorce who wants to have cosmetic surgery to get back at a spouse. There are also those patients who think surgery will change their life or make them happier. Or the person who believes that if his nose were a little smaller, he would be more successful or have women falling for him. These scenarios are a set up for a disappointed patient. Sometimes I can foresee this problem, and sometimes I can't. The most difficult patients to read are the quiet ones. They come into the consultation with very few questions. Their minds are already made up, and suddenly they are ready to schedule surgery, even when I may not have decided whether I am comfortable operating on them. Every plastic surgeon has come across patients who are obviously unbalanced. The best approach in these situations is to simply say, "I don't think I can help you." Cosmetic surgery changes the outside, but it does not change the person on the inside.

Baby boomers are getting older; one boomer turns 60 every six seconds. They are determined not to grow old before their time. This quest for eternal youth has spawned the proliferation of medi-spas, anti-aging clinics, Botox® emporiums, and cosmeceutical brands. This trend is here to stay and we can expect a wave of new developments in the near future.

A Commitment to Excellence has its Rewards

My advice to those considering plastic surgery as a career is to work hard, be ethical, and honest, don't oversell, and don't hesitate to tell a patient that he doesn't' need a procedure if that is what you really believe. Taking the long view of my practice, that advice has paid off many times over. I tell people, don't do this; you don't need it; you are not ready. They may not book their surgery now, but they send their friends to me because they are impressed with my integrity, and I know they will come back to me when the time is right.

I feel very fortunate to be part of the specialty of plastic surgery. I love what I do, I look forward to coming to work every day, and I hope that enthusiasm translates to my staff, patients and colleagues. It is very rewarding on a personal level to be able to deliver the improvements patients seek, to see the smiles on their faces and their renewed sense of self-esteem. You can make your living in any number of ways, but there is perhaps more diversity in plastic surgery than in any other medical or surgical specialty. You never get bored, and every day brings new challenges. Plastic surgery is a constantly evolving specialty that is only limited by a surgeon's imagination and creativity.

Barry J. Cohen, M.D., P.C. is a fully trained plastic and reconstructive surgeon. He practices all areas of plastic and reconstructive surgery, with areas of greatest interest in cosmetic surgery.

Dr. Cohen's educational background is broad. He is a graduate of Cornell University with a Bachelor of Arts in Biochemistry. While at Cornell, Dr. Cohen was involved in the honors program in his major. He completed his medical school training at Georgetown University, graduating near the top of his class. He then served as a general surgery resident at the well known local trauma center, The Washington Hospital Center, where he won numerous awards for both his clinical and research skills. His plastic surgery training was taken in New York with The Long Island Plastic Surgical Group. The Long Island Plastic Surgical group is comprised of the largest group of plastic surgeons in the world, exposing Dr. Cohen to all facets of plastic surgery. Besides his broad clinical training, Dr. Cohen has published numerous articles in the field of plastic surgery.

His current hospital affiliations include: Suburban Hospital, Shady Grove Hospital, Sibley Hospital, Holy Cross Hospital, Montgomery General Hospital, and The Washington Hospital Center. He also has privileges at The Montgomery Surgery Center.

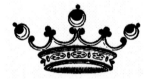

Plastic Surgery for a New Millennium

Jay M. Pensler, M.D.

Associate Professor, Clinical Plastic Surgery
Northwestern University Medical School

The Art and Science of Plastic Surgery

Plastic surgery is a discipline that deals with modification of face and body features through the molding and remodeling of soft tissue. "Plastic" is an ancient Greek term that originally meant "fit for molding." The art of plastic surgery is similar to sculpting or other types of art where you assess three-dimensional aspects of a problem and provide a solution. Plastic surgery seeks to optimize form and function, yet it differs significantly from art in that there is a fourth dimension which must be considered: the patient.

The science of plastic surgery involves a great deal of research. New developments in the materials and instruments that we use have radically changed how plastic surgery is performed. We are able to do more while being less invasive because of advances made in the scientific side of the field. I would expect the technical advances to accelerate further changes over the next ten to fifteen years.

The Surgeon's Role

Each patient comes with his or her own unique set of surgical and psychological issues. A surgeon needs to sort through those issues and determine if a patient's problems can be solved or the situation improved. If the answer is yes, the surgeon must then assess a variety of options, all the while balancing risks and benefits, before determining what the optimal solution is for that particular patient. Also, the surgeon needs to take into consideration the patient's expectation for improvement, patient costs and recovery time.

The Path to Becoming a Plastic Surgeon

To become a successful plastic surgeon you need good fundamental medical knowledge attained through education at a reputable medical school. One of your goals should be a residency at a top-rated institution where you will have an opportunity to work with quality individuals. You also need to complete a board certification procedure, which includes a written educational component as well as a practice evaluation component where you present cases and assess them for quality control. After completing these steps, you can then claim to be a board-certified plastic surgeon. When you are starting out in practice, the likelihood of successfully treating a complex problem is significantly less than after you have treated similar problems. You need a great deal of experience in a wide range of circumstances to determine your capabilities. When you have about ten years of independent experience you will have acquired the skills and knowledge necessary to treat a wide range of patients in your practice in a highly reproducible manner.

The previous statement should not be construed to mean that individuals finishing their training are not ready to treat patients; nothing could be further from the truth. The point is that to perform a complex surgical procedure there is no substitute for high quality experience. If someone has performed a procedure five hundred times incorrectly, the five hundred and first time it is performed it will most likely be sub-optimal. If an individual is well trained and has performed the procedure correctly five hundred times, the predictability of a successful outcome is obviously enhanced but never guaranteed.

You can choose many directions within plastic surgery. These include hand surgery, cosmetic surgery, microsurgery, reconstructive surgery and craniofacial surgery. In addition, there is a pediatric component to plastic surgery.

As far as skills are concerned, you must have good hand-eye coordination to produce surgical results with a high degree of predictability. One of the most important criteria for being a successful plastic surgeon is the desire to be a perfectionist. In the operating room, you can't be afraid to redo a procedure several times until it is done correctly. How quickly you perform the surgery is not as important as the final results. Highly successful plastic surgeons display a determination and tenacity to stay with the case until it is absolutely perfect given the pre-existing anatomy.

The Patient's Initial Visit

Communication with plastic surgery patients occurs on several levels. Office staff is the first point of contact for plastic surgery patients. For this reason, I spend a lot of time educating my staff so that they can communicate better with patients.

In most instances, I spend an hour with a patient when discussing aesthetic problems. The first part of a visit usually focuses on the individual's medical history. You need to determine if the patient is healthy or if there are any problems, which could pose a surgical risk.

During the second part of the visit, patient and doctor can discuss what is perceived to be the problem. This is also a good time for taking photographs of the particular area or areas involved. By viewing the photographs on a computer screen and using digital imaging, we can give the patient a clear picture of how things look before surgery and what they may look like afterward. I think patients also find it helpful to see photographs of others with similar problems so that they will have a realistic idea of what to expect from the surgery.

If a patient is requesting a procedure with which I don't have significant experience, I will send them to a doctor who has more skill in that area. You always want to offer the patient a highly predictable outcome based on the parameters of their problem. One of my mentors offered me a great piece of advice: If you treat every patient as you would a member of your family, you will be very busy and your patients will be very happy. The goal is to achieve the optimal result for your patient, not to see how many individual surgeries you can perform.

Psychological Factors

Between 1997 and 2002, the number of cosmetic surgeries performed in the United States saw an increase of roughly 228 percent. The majority of my practice is cosmetic surgery, also referred to as aesthetic surgery. In addition to an increase in the number of individuals who want plastic surgery, we are also seeing a larger cross-section of society seeking this type of surgery. America is still the great melting pot and as our society has become more diverse so have plastic surgeons' practices.

As more people opt for surgery, you find more people who are not candidates for the procedure due to psychological reasons. Plastic surgeons must spend a great deal of time with each individual prior to surgery to determine the patient's mental stability and psychological readiness for the procedure. If you get a sense that the patient is unstable, surgery should not be recommended. It can be extremely difficult, if not impossible, to identify a determined individual who has decided they need to have something done.

Keeping Up-to-Date with Technology

Plastic surgery is a field that is actively changing. You have to do a lot of reading and talking with colleagues about what is new and in development. If there is a new technique you are interested in, it's helpful to visit colleagues who are practicing the technique so that you can learn from them

Sometimes procedures once considered popular begin causing late problems for patients. Ongoing evaluation of procedures, instruments and products is key if a plastic surgeon wants to offer patients the latest in surgical advances. Our patients depend on us for sorting through the maze of new products and procedures.

Self Evaluation and Success

The best plastic surgeons are their own worst critic. You have to continually evaluate each result and assess operating room procedures, instruments and techniques.

Each patient presents a unique set of challenges. Every time you finish with a case, you need to honestly assess how well you solved the patient's problem. You will then be in a better position to address the same problem when it presents itself in a different patient. Improvement comes from a combination of critical thinking and the ability to make necessary changes; it is a constant evolution.

In plastic surgery, there are many measurements of success; of these, patient satisfaction is paramount. Recognition by one's colleagues is also a positive, but the end result for the patient is most important. We're able to offer a patient a solution that may allow them to live their life in a totally different way. The fact that we can be part of altering – in a significant and positive manner – the way someone perceives him or herself is tremendously rewarding.

There are several different venues in which a plastic surgeon can gain recognition. In the clinical arena, the operation itself – and the surgical skill that it requires – is viewed as the most important part of this field. Some individuals, however, spend very little time operating and focus on research and/or resident education instead. There are still others who focus both on clinical skills and research. Whether you are a great surgeon or a great researcher, you can positively affect a large number of individuals. You can become a leader in the plastic surgery field either through clinical practice or research, or both.

Experience makes the difference between a plastic surgeon being good and great. Great surgeons are also characterized by the following: good three-dimensional skills, critical thinking and innovation. To be truly outstanding in the field, you have to continually innovate, write, publish, and evaluate your performance

Changes and Trends

Today, we are seeing an increase in the non-surgical alternatives we can offer patients. For example, we can inject fillers and paralyze muscles much more effectively than we could years ago. There are some new fillers being tried in Canada and Europe that may prove worthwhile. Those new technologies may be available in the United States in the future. As a surgeon, you need to be knowledgeable about alternatives to surgery in order to offer patients an array of treatments that will achieve the best possible outcome.

Surgical techniques and instrumentation also have changed dramatically in recent years. We increasingly rely on very small incisions and minimal invasive surgery. We use more specialized instruments, such as endoscopes, which eliminate the need for very large incisions. The technology available to surgeons is continually changing. You need to keep up with the changes and assess how they can enhance your practice and the results your patients get.

There have been many changes in medicine during the past 20 to 30 years that have been negative. The issue of third party payers and insurance companies continues to put a great deal of stress on medical practices, particularly in regard to paperwork and reimbursement. Insurance companies try to pit patients against doctors. This has made the practice of medicine more difficult for both physicians and patients.

A Promising Field

Some plastic surgeons are very meticulous and others are not. In any specialty there is always a wide spectrum of talent and skill; plastic surgery is no exception. Plastic surgeons must be interested with form and function, and they must have the capacity to see problems three-dimensionally. The ability to balance artistic ability and science is essential in this field.

When dealing with patients, it is best to under promise and over deliver. Always, you need to be realistic about the results you can achieve. Being very fair and honest with your patients is, by far, the best approach.

This specialty continues to be the focus of a great deal of research on a number of fronts. In the future, I think we will see an increase in non-surgical cosmetic procedures. As new methods become available, those that hold the most promise and prove most effective will be incorporated into daily practice. The field of plastic surgery is always changing, and we are always exploring. It is a fascinating journey that we are all taking.

Dr. Jay Michael Pensler obtained his M.D. from the University of Chicago Pritzker School of Medicine in 1980 and his M.B.A. from Northwestern University in 1995. Dr. Pensler studied plastic surgery at the University of Texas Medical Branch. He served as a general surgery resident at the New York University Medical Center and studied craniofacial surgery at Harvard University.

Dr. Pensler is the associate professor of Clinical Plastic Surgery at Northwestern University Medical School. He is affiliated with Northwestern Memorial Hospital Chicago, Evanston Northwestern Healthcare, and Children's Memorial Hospital.

Dedication *– For my wife and kids, Laurie, Arielle and Alexander*

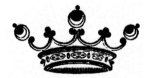

The Successful Plastic Surgeon

Lance G. Leithauser, M.D.

Board Certified Plastic Surgeon
Shady Grove Center for Plastic, Cosmetic and
Reconstructive Surgery

Becoming a Successful Plastic Surgeon

There are many different qualities required to be a successful plastic surgeon: intelligence, good eye-hand coordination and people skills are certainly all important. I would say the two most important skills are communications skills and artistic judgment. The ability to use each of these skills at the time and place they are required is the key to success.

Artistic judgment may sound odd initially, but plastic surgery is really a blend of art and science. Art is essential because you have to be able to envision the desired result before surgery begins. That determines which operation is chosen and how it is performed. The scientific aspect is the more typical medical knowledge — anatomy, biology, pharmacology, and in the case of lasers, physics. A good plastic surgeon combines artistic ability and scientific knowledge to produce the desired result for each individual patient.

I think that a great plastic surgeon is someone who can get good results in difficult cases. Anyone can get good results from an easy case, but the ability to get even a fair result in a very difficult case is the mark of a great plastic surgeon.

The most challenging aspect of being a plastic surgeon is dealing with unrealistic or unattainable desires of some patients. Every surgeon wants to please the patient, but sometimes it is not possible. The only thing you can do is to try to see where the patient is coming from, but you have to temper that with the reality that you can't satisfy everyone. Still, it's always a disappointment.

Litigious patients are another very difficult aspect of the job. What I try to do to deal with those people is to keep communication open as much as possible. They are getting advice from their attorney, who is not encouraging communication with my office. I also try to remember that the vast majority of patients are happy with my work.

Training

Of course, you have to graduate from medical school first. After you graduate from medical school, you'll do a residency. Most plastic surgeons will go through general surgery residency, which is anywhere from three to six years. Some plastic surgery residents will go through an ear, nose, and throat residency or occasionally orthopedic or another residency first, but the bulk of them will go through general surgery. Then you have plastic surgery training for two to three years and that will vary from area to area. Some people then take a fellowship for six months if they have a specific field of interest such as cosmetics or microsurgery. It's a long road with many years of training before you're certified.

Training continues once you're practicing as well. There are lots of changes in this field, so you have to stay current. There are lots of ways to stay on top of the industry knowledge. I like to go to meetings often, and I read the journals every month. I frequently discuss new developments with my colleagues. By far, the best way to learn the skills for plastic surgery is good residency training. If you have good training as a resident and good preparation, you can go out and learn new things as they come and adapt to it well. If you don't have good training, you're always sort of behind the pack.

Patient Care

At my office we try to give good patient service, as well as good patient care. Any plastic surgeon would try to provide good care to give the best operation, the best materials, the best possible surgery, but I think that good service is also very important in my area. That means returning phone calls promptly and keeping time in the waiting room to a minimum. Most people don't respond well to prolonged waits. The best way to communicate with patients by far is face to face. If we can't do that, we'll call them. Emails or written letters are much less personal. I think the single most important thing for communication is to leave enough time to answer patients' questions. If they are feeling rushed, they are not going to feel that's good communication.

When a patient comes in for a consultation, I consider the aspects of that person's specific case. Each situation varies, depending on what the problem is. Some people will come in with minor problems: they'll want a mole or cyst or something small removed. For cases like that, we'll talk to them and get a medical history and make sure there are no underlying medical problems. We'll examine the patient to see what the problem is, discuss with them how we do the surgery and then eventually schedule the surgery.

For complicated cases, for example breast implants or a facelift, you have to give a lot more detail with options of different ways to do the operation. For breast implants, you can use smooth implants or textured implants, you can put them above the pectoral muscle or below it. You can make your incision nearly indistinct underneath the breast. Different patients will heal in different ways, so we don't do it the same way every time. Each approach has advantages and disadvantages and what might be a disadvantage to one patient might be less of a concern to another. You weigh all of those factors and choose the best operation for them. It would take a lot more time to do a work up like that.

Risk is also an issue that I discuss thoroughly with each patient, though it's a very broad subject because it is associated with a specific surgery. For minor procedures, such as removing a cyst or a mole, the risk might consist only of minor pain. But for major operations, there is a large range of potential problems, depending on the scope of the individual operation.

It's important to discuss all the options and aspects of an operation fully because some people have misconceptions about what we can and cannot do. Many people will say that they came to a plastic surgeon because they don't want any scars. You have to explain that it's impossible to do surgery without scars and that the scars will be permanent. You can take time and care to minimize those scars by being careful. I think it's more of a willingness and ability to take the time to line things up the best you can.

Finding the Right Doctor

I'm a believer in good residency training, so I think that board certification is a very important criterion to look for. Then you know that the surgeon has not only been through an accredited program, but also has passed a two-part series of tests to become certified. I think this acts as sort of a background check to some extent. It tells you that this person has proper training and has passed a complex system of tests to prove it. I think that's the single most important thing in finding a plastic surgeon.

Hopes for the Future

These are kind of turbulent times. Managed care has made it difficult to get some reconstructive operations covered for patients. Another problem has been the changes in malpractice insurance. These changes have made it difficult in some parts of the country for doctors to afford or even obtain malpractice insurance. I'm an optimist, though I recognize that there are problems with insurance –

the biggest problem being that 40 million people don't even have insurance. I do believe that these things can be worked out and I have no doubt that in ten or twenty years that we'll have dedicated, hard working plastic surgeons doing our job.

I'd also like to see some new drugs on the market. As a plastic surgeon, the most valuable new drug in my work would be a local anesthetic that you could just rub on the skin so that people wouldn't have to get shots. Patients are always asking, "Don't you have something you can just spray on or rub on?" We have to tell them no, they have to have a shot. So that would be a very valuable product if it worked consistently and effectively.

Advice

Always try to be professional and courteous. For me, what is important is providing the best patient care and the best patient service that I can give day after day. Satisfaction comes from achieving good results and having satisfied patients. That's when I feel best about my job and good about myself. Also, I have a family with five children. It has always been more important to me to have more family time and less practice time. Some of my colleagues do not have a family or they have a smaller family, so it's different for them.

The golden rules for a plastic surgeon would be similar to the golden rules of life: to determine what your patient needs and do your best to fulfill those needs.

Lance G. Leithauser served as a general surgeon resident at Georgetown University Hospital. He worked for two years at West Penn Hospital before establishing a practice at the Shady Grove Center for Plastic, Cosmetic and Reconstructive Surgery. He has served as chairman of the board for the Department of Plastic Surgery for the Greater Laurel-Beltsville Hospital and HealthSouth Montgomery Surgical Center and as vice chairman for Shady Grove Adventist Hospital. Dr. Leithauser is board certified in plastic surgery. He received his BA from Swarthmore College in 1969 and his MD from the University of Michigan Medical School in 1973.

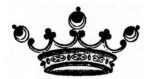

Focusing on the Patient

A. Dean Jabs, M.D., Ph.D., FACS &
Franklin D. Richards, M.D., FACS

Board Certified Plastic Surgeons
Cosmetic Surgery Associates

Seeing the Whole Picture

The science of plastic surgery is a blend of medicine and surgery with engineering and art.

The art of being a plastic surgeon is being able to interpret the physical changes a patient requests with the image they see in the mirror, which is governed by more than just their physical appearance. It is being able to relate the psychological status of the patient with how they see themselves. Many of the physical changes we make have a profound psychological effect. Being able to discern what a patient says they want and what their real motivations are come with experience.

As a plastic surgeon, you don't treat strictly flesh, blood, and bone. There is also a very large emotional and psychological component of your work. Part of the art of plastic surgery is being able to define and understand what the patient truly wants. Your job is to listen to what they are telling you, certainly, but you must understand them emotionally in the context of their entire humanity.

The Psychology of Plastic Surgery

The role of a plastic surgeon is to discern our patients' goals, desires, and expectations, match them with what we can offer, and devise the appropriate procedures to accomplish the process.

Plastic surgery is not merely beauty surgery. A plastic surgeon interacts with patients who have had trauma or cancer and have lost body parts. The plastic surgeon tries to make patients whole by restoring their bodies – even in some cases of cosmetic surgery: You restore their bodies to what they see with their inner eye, and that sometimes gives them an entirely different outlook on life.

There are certain patients who come in for procedures on whom you don't want to operate because what they are asking for surgically does not match with what they are asking for psychologically. The only possible outcome is that you will never match the patient's expectations with the surgical procedure.

For instance, if a woman whose husband has left her for a younger woman comes to you and says she wants to look younger, what she actually wants is her husband back. You can make her look great, but if her husband does not return, in her mind the reason is obviously that the surgery has failed.

Quality of Training and Patient Care

Plastic surgery requires years of training – four years of college, four years of medical school followed by six to seven years of residency. Along with training come testing requirements and boards that have been established to help distinguish those physicians who have met certain knowledge and surgical skill requirements sufficiently to be called board-certified.

A plastic surgeon not only has to be knowledgeable with the field and be a good technical surgeon, but also has to work well with people. As we mentioned earlier, you frequently have to be able to read between the lines with patients in identifying and understanding what the patient wants and what the patient needs. Many problems have no clear-cut answers. You are often called upon to use mature judgment to make decisions that will be best for the patient.

A very important rule in plastic surgery is that the patient comes first, no matter what. As long as you remember that, all of the other aspects of the art and science fit into place.

Plastic surgeons do cosmetic surgery. All doctors who do cosmetic surgery are not necessarily plastic surgeons. We are sometimes asked to testify as expert witnesses. I (Dr. Richards) testified recently in a case against a gynecologist who performed liposuction with disastrous effects. The gynecologist had learned to do liposuction by taking a one-week course in Europe and then came back and started doing the procedure.

As plastic surgeons, that casualness about our specialty is foreign to us. Those types of procedures are an integral part of our training that took years to master. The thought of taking a week-long course, returning to the States, and practicing unsupervised is appalling.

Patients trust physicians and believe they will be well cared for and given a quality product when they go to any physician. That is sadly not necessarily true. Patients need to do their homework. Many people call themselves plastic surgeons or confuse the public by stating they are cosmetic surgeons.

If someone is going to have plastic surgery, the first thing to do is to check out the physician and get personal references from friends or family members. Then the patient should schedule an appointment to meet with the physician to discuss needs and objectives to meet them. If the patient cannot relate to the physician on a comfortable, human level, another physician should be sought.

Ideal Communication Channel with Patients

Before we do any surgical procedure, a patient typically makes more than one office visit, each of which can last from half an hour to an hour or longer. We talk about the patient's goals and desires, and we talk about what we can possibly achieve.

Most of our discussion is verbal. Sometimes, however, our office staff will pick up clues in talking to patients about information that they sense the patient may not have passed on to the physician. These clues, these bits of information, will help us know and understand the patient a little better.

We also have technologies that help us communicate with the patient. Computerized imaging systems allow us to digitize photos of the patient, perform virtual surgery, and show the patient what the results could look like after surgery.

When a patient has doubt, it is usually because of lack of information. We then try to define what they are missing and supply it. Sometimes they don't understand what you are saying; other times they have read something on the Internet, or they've heard a friend say something erroneous, or they have read something that is correct but did not understand it.

When patients doubt facts, we have to straighten out the facts for them. If they doubt our results, we have to show them the results they can obtain and the facts. With some patients, we have to be sure we are on top of our game and able to quote the journal articles, and we have to ask them about what is actually bothering them.

Diagnostic and Planning Processes

For a cosmetic procedure, a patient usually obtains our name from a friend, the Internet, a phone book, or a referral from another physician. During the first appointment, we take a history and go over some of the goals they want to achieve. This is when we begin to know the patient as we talk about lifestyle, jobs, hobbies, and family. We also discuss their expectations.

The examination concentrates on the areas a patient is concerned about changing. Then we make recommendations on these areas, as well as others we feel should be enhanced also if they relate to those concerns. For example, a man might come to us believing he wants a smaller nose. When we examine him, however, we find it's not his nose that's too big, but his chin that's too small, and we can show him how enlarging his chin will resolve his concern of a large nose.

After the examination is complete and recommendations are made, the patient talks with our patient care coordinator. The procedures are reviewed again, and prices are discussed. The patient is then left with the decision of whether or not to pursue the surgery. Very often patients will have additional questions or concerns and will come back for a second or third visit before making a decision.

For reconstructive surgery consultations, we are usually consulted by another physician for a problem they have, and the consultation is very problem-focused. The first concern is to evaluate the condition of the patient and get specifics on what the consulting physician is asking us to do. Sometimes the problem is wide open, such as broken facial bones from a motor vehicle accident. Other times it is very focused, like reconstruction of the breast because of the effects of breast cancer treatment.

We need to make sure the patient is in good enough shape to undergo any surgery we plan. We also need to find out the mental status of the patient. We have to determine whether there are family members involved because they will be part of the decision-making process.

Once those points are covered, we mentally make a checklist of possible ways to fix the problem. Most plastic surgeons set this up as a reconstructive ladder in their minds, starting with the simplest way to fix the problem and working the way up the ladder to more complex types of procedures, always weighing the risks and benefits of each. Every decision in medicine is a risk/benefit ratio.

When we come across the procedure that has the lowest risk with the highest benefit, that is usually the one we tell the patient we want to do. But we always make sure we have what we call a "lifeboat," or an alternative plan. If the plan we have made does not work, we need to have another plan we can fall back on. One of the cardinal rules is to make sure plan A is not the same as plan B.

Clearly, the major consideration in plastic surgery – and this is true for all surgery – is that the surgeon's ego truly doesn't matter. What matters is the patient's well being. If you have a complication with a patient or if you are in a situation where you feel as though you are getting in over your head, you need to ask for help. There is no shame in asking for help. The shame is in *not* asking for help when you need it.

Challenges for Plastic Surgeons

Striking a balance between our personal and professional lives is a constant challenge in any professional's life. Everyone has a comfort level with how much time they spend in the profession and how much time they spend with their family. It is probably generally more healthful to spend a little more time with your family than we all do, not only for our own sanity and emotional well being, but for the benefit of our patients, as well.

If there is a problem, it is that we are all driven, Type A personalities who are anal retentive on getting our jobs done and not missing anything. Almost anyone who is a success in business is that way. Everyone has to look inside and find the balance that feels right.

The most challenging aspect of plastic surgery is knowing what application or what new development to apply to a problem. As each innovation is introduced, you don't want to be the first person on the bandwagon to use it, but neither do you want to be the last. The greatest challenge is knowing how to approach those problems with the new knowledge we gain.

Measuring Success

As physicians, we measure success by how happy we can make each patient. It's tempting sometimes to try to do a procedure on a patient just because it can be done, but it may not necessarily be what will make the patient happy. If we can make the patient happy and feel satisfied that they have had a worthwhile experience, then we have been successful. It may mean that no surgery is done. Whatever is best for the patient is what will make us good physicians. The ultimate way to measure success is for your patient to be happy.

A well performed procedure that you are happy with and that achieves the patient's goals with as little downtime and risk as possible in the most time effective and cost effective manner is another way to measure success.

Respecting Other Surgeons

What impresses us about other plastic surgeons is how willing they are to share their experience and how good their results are.

Leaders in our national society are usually individuals who have published many journal articles or who are heads of academic programs. Those people have sought leadership opportunities and relationships and friendships with people who help them attain positions and offices in our national society.

There are also leaders in our local community or local medical society. Attaining these positions requires building good relationships with other physicians, as well as good relationships and a solid reputation among patients. Those kinds of strengths will make a surgeon a leader in the local community without having to get involved in the politics of being a leader in national organizations.

From Good to Better to Best

Once you have completed your residency and become a plastic surgeon, what it takes to be a good one is being cautious and thinking of patient safety first. Look for help and direction from others who have been around longer.

A surgeon who uses good judgment, who listens to his or her patients, who tries to help them achieve their goals, and who is seriously concerned about the patient as the center of the entire experience will be a successful surgeon. Someone who seeks growth in his or her medical knowledge and who stays up-to-date on relevant technologies is likely to be very successful.

A great plastic surgeon stays current, and cannot get stagnant. Attaining this level usually also requires experience.

Innovation, the ability to see the possible and to do the impossible, is what separates a good plastic surgeon from a great one. Being able to take the next step and having the courage to do so as someone who logically thinks things through and sees a possibility for taking the science and the art to the next level elevates a good plastic surgeon to a great plastic surgeon.

Changes and Trends in Plastic Surgery

Over the last five to ten years, the medical marketplace has increased pressure on surgeons to do more cosmetic surgery than reconstructive surgery – a big change. There is increased competition at all levels from both other plastic surgeons and those who want to be plastic surgeons. Most people have no idea what a plastic surgeon is, nor do they have a real understanding of cosmetic surgery. People think there is something called a board-certified cosmetic surgeon, but there is no such thing.

Also within the field of surgery, advances we have seen over the last 20 years push us toward less invasive procedures that can achieve the same results with faster recovery. That has been pushing the specialty, as well.

Changes over the next five to ten years will include the field becoming more crowded. As the baby boomers age, we'll have more and more people seeking elective surgery. We will see more technology involved as computers continue to play a more important role in surgery. They are used extensively in imaging now. Perhaps we'll be able to use that imaging technology somehow to scan contours of people's faces and use the results to determine how to augment or reduce bone or fat to change the way patients look.

We can see the possibility in the future of using fetal tissue. Even now we can make cells differentiate to fetal tissues, which have the potential to become almost anything. Once that becomes accepted practice, it will become a viable alternative to using fetal cells, opening wide a door to the possibility of growing new limbs or other body parts to replace those that have been severed because of trauma or disease.

We would like to see technology that would allow us to control scarring. There has been some research in fetal tissue. Fetuses don't scar; they heal without forming a scar. It would be wonderful to discover how adults might heal without scarring.

Keeping up with Technology

New advances in plastic surgery are constantly being made. The field's knowledge continues to grow exponentially. As physicians, we keep on top of what is going on by reading journals. We subscribe to several monthlies that report comprehensively on research.

Our professional associations keep us informed of relevant news on a regular basis over the Internet. We also receive information from our state medical societies, as well as our national societies in the form of emails and articles and journals, but also in meetings. We can attend several meetings a year to learn about and discuss new advances, new achievements, and new techniques in plastic surgery.

The plastic surgery specialty is broad: Someone once said plastic surgery is surgery of the skin and its contents. We are one of the few specialties that operate on the body literally from head to toe. It takes a great deal of effort and time to remain current in this field.

Some things don't change. Medical literature from years ago will offer advice that is equally applicable today: Listen to your patient; your patient will tell you the diagnosis, and you can move forward together. That advice applies in plastic surgery, too.

A. Dean Jabs, M.D., Ph.D., FACS:

Dr. A. Dean Jabs is a board certified, internationally recognized plastic surgeon dedicated to providing quality, state of the art plastic surgery to patients in the Washington, DC metro area as well as to patients from around the world. He has been in practice since 1989 and possesses skills that draw plastic surgeons from around the country to observe his surgeries. Dr. Jabs has a special interest in facial rejuvenation, breast augmentation and nasal surgery (rhinoplasty). Dr. Jabs is noted for his warm, personal demeanor and a passion for the details of cosmetic surgery that lead to extraordinary results. Establishing a personal relationship that allows him to understand his patients concerns and desires is a key part of his consultation process. His outgoing personality and his outstanding surgical skill have led many local physicians and their families to seek his care.

Dr. Jabs is a leader in his field. He has been elected President of the National Capital Society of Plastic Surgeons by his local plastic surgery colleagues where he previously served as Secretary and Vice-President of the society. At the national level Dr. Jabs serves on the International Committee of the American Society for Aesthetic Plastic Surgery. Dr. Jabs was selected by the Consumer Research Council of America as one of America's Top Surgeons. He is listed in America's Cosmetic Doctors Consumer Guide and has been featured in articles in The Potomac Gazette as well as Plastic Surgery News. He has also appeared in The Washingtonian magazine.

He is Board Certified by the American Board of Plastic Surgery and is a Fellow of the American College of Surgeons (FACS). He is also a member of the American Society of Plastic Surgeons, The American Society for Aesthetic Plastic Surgery and the Northeastern Society of Plastic Surgeons. He holds the prestigious Certificate of Added Qualification in Cosmetic Surgery from the American Society of

Aesthetic Plastic Surgery (ASAPS) as well as the Physicians Recognition Award from the American Medical Association.

Dr. Jabs graduated from the University of Southern California before pursuing graduate work at the University of Illinois in Chicago where he received a Ph.D. in Immunology. He then attended Rush Medical College in Chicago obtaining his M.D. in 1984. Dr. Jabs trained in general surgery at St. Vincent's Hospital in New York City followed by plastic surgery training at world renowned Columbia University before moving to the Washington, D.C. area.

Dr. Jabs has authored several papers on plastic surgery topics and has presented at major national meetings of plastic surgeons. He is on staff at Suburban Hospital in Maryland and Fairfax Hospital in Virginia. He is an Assistant Clinical Professor of Surgery at the Uniformed Services University of the Health Sciences in Bethesda and has held academic appointments at the University of Connecticut and at Columbia University in New York .

Franklin D. Richards, M.D., FACS:

A long-standing resident of the Washington D.C. metro area and a graduate of George Washington University in 1982, Dr. Franklin Richards, M.D., is board certified and has been in practice fourteen years, possessing cosmetic surgical expertise that draws plastic surgeons from around the country to observe his techniques. Dr. Richards specializes in facial procedures, breast augmentation, liposuction and body contouring.

Patients who meet with Dr. Richards immediately recognize both the passion he has for his work and the professional manner in which he deals with people. The concerns and goals of the patient are principal in forming his thoughtful and honest evaluations. His outstanding abilities inspire such confidence that fellow doctors and their spouses, when in need of cosmetic procedures, come to Dr. Richards. His surgical skill, trustworthiness and approachability have earned him a lasting reputation.

Voted President of the National Capital Society of Plastic Surgeons in 2002, Dr. Richards has assumed a leadership role in his field. He has presented at national meetings and been published in national professional journals. He has been the recipient of the Physicians Recognition Award from the American Medical Association (AMA) and the prestigious Certificate of Advanced Education in Cosmetic Surgery from the American Society for Aesthetic Plastic Surgery (ASAPS). Dr. Richards is cited in the National Consumer Checkbook 'Top Doctor List' and the National Consumer Research Council of America has listed him as one of 'America's Top Surgeons.'

Dr. Richards' skill and expertise have also been established locally. Washingtonian magazine has recognized him in their 'Top Plastic Surgeons' list, and has done so since 1995. His expert opinion has been sought by numerous prominent publications, including The Washington Post and Washingtonian magazine.

As a Fellow of the American College of Surgeons (FACS) and a member of several distinguished surgical associations, including the American Society of Plastic Surgeons (ASPS) and the American Society for Aesthetic Plastic Surgery (ASAPS), Dr. Richards continues to avail himself of the collective knowledge and progress in fields of plastic and cosmetic surgery.

Dr. Richards was privileged to have served his country as an attending plastic surgeon at Walter Reed Army Medical Center in Washington, DC. He also served as director of the Burn Unit at William Beaumont Army Medical Center during Desert Storm I.

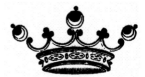

Understanding the Aesthetic Plastic Surgeon

Mark E. Richards, M.D.
Board Certified Plastic Surgeon
Ageless Impressions Plastic Surgery Institute

Behind the Veil of a Plastic Surgeon: An Individual's Approach to Art and Science

Simply put, the art and science of plastic surgery involves making physical improvements to a fellow human being so that that person is able to meet a higher aesthetic or functional standard. As a plastic surgeon, I try to blend my scientific and technical knowledge with a creative aesthetic and artistic spirit in order to transform my clients' suboptimal features into pleasing and functional ones. In success, this physical transformation often causes marked improvements in their emotional and psychological outlook. While this marked change in outlook seems unusual to the casual observer, how we look to ourselves strongly effects how we project to others and, reflectively, how they treat us in return.

Aesthetics

After plastic surgery, the results may be beautiful in some cases, while in others it may mean achieving a normal to mildly attractive appearance. The goal is to achieve a satisfying improvement in the areas of surgical change that integrates with the person's looks in untreated areas. Ethnic and familial characteristics must be considered in an effort not to create a bizarre appearance. Evaluation of the client involves understanding how the undesirable features can be changed to compliment the existing desirable features so that the whole is greater in aesthetic beauty than the sum of the individual parts. We are improving form and function. Functional improvement could mean socially functional (e.g. more accepted or sought after), utilitarian functionality (such as having clothing fit better), or mechanically functional (such as improved nasal airflow). Sometimes, the functional improvement involves all three aspects.

Science

The science involved in becoming a plastic surgeon involves developing a deep understanding of anatomy, biochemistry and physiology, as well as training in the core curriculum of surgical fundamentals such as wound healing. Usually plastic surgeons obtain that type of knowledge during college and medical school (8 years), 4 to 5 years of general surgery training, and 2 to 3 years of plastic surgery training. Despite what is typically 10 or 11 years of post-college training and education, this specialized training teaches only the basic fundamentals, goals, and principles of plastic surgery. From there, one begins a plastic surgery "practice" and adapts these fundamental principles to meet and solve the ever changing challenges which arise.

Elements Necessary for Success as a Plastic Surgeon

There are three necessary (though not sufficient in themselves) elements to becoming successful as a plastic surgeon. I believe this holds true regardless of how you define success, unless the only yard stick you are using is wealth.

The first attribute involves being an observer and diagnostician. The plastic surgeon must understand through accurate observation and evaluation the real deficiencies and problems that exist for that patient. He must also understand the patient's own perception of their "deficiencies."

The second attribute of a plastic surgeon is that of innovator. It is important that a plastic surgeon not only provides treatment, but also develops innovative techniques and personalized responses to different problems. This creative role is the responsibility that makes plastic surgery unique within the field of medicine. Many of the current improved results from aesthetic plastic surgery are based upon our ever deepening appreciation of anatomy as it relates to how the external form is affected by the changes associated with aging or trauma.

The third attribute is one of being an educator. The surgeon needs to communicate to the patient his or her treatment options, as well as reasonable expectations regarding the outcome, potential risks and potential complications. While we like to think of plastic surgery as limitless in potential, this is not the case. Because of the large variations in the pre-existing conditions of clients, the successful plastic surgeon must have the ability to decide what realistic post-surgical results are possible and desirable. This must then be communicated clearly.

Qualities of a Successful Plastic Surgeon

The successful plastic surgeon will display several notable qualities, the first one among them being empathy. This quality is an important requirement for any physician. If you cannot empathize with the patient's concerns and feelings, you will not be able to adequately understand what needs to be done to help them.

Another quality, more specific to plastic surgery, would be aesthetic creativity. Each plastic surgery patient's problems are uniquely different. The surgical approach must be individualized for each patient to get the most ideal results. If you approach a plastic surgery procedure as merely a technical exercise, you end up performing the same procedure for everyone with similar "problems." This will lead to results that are less than ideal.

A related attribute would be intellectual curiosity. There can be no ideal procedure or ideal result. The best a great plastic surgeon is able to do is to utilize his finest techniques in order to give the best possible result he can at that point in time. The best plastic surgeons always try to improve, and see each result not as a triumph, but as a source of satisfaction and education as to what can be changed to make the next result even better.

Tenaciousness, as demonstrated by tenacity of purpose, is another necessary ingredient. You must be willing to "stick to it." Plastic surgery involves a long formal training process, followed by a lifelong process of educating yourself after training. All of which requires tremendous energy and effort.

In order to stay on top in this field, it helps to have an artist's love of beauty. Appreciation of the beauty of form and function is what keeps us striving to be better and develop new techniques.

Another important attribute is "good hands." This is the ability to sense through your fingers what the tissues are doing, what they are willing to do and what they are not able to do. This essentially is a "sixth sense" through your fingertips.

Finally, a successful plastic surgeon must be humble. Doctors are not God and the world does not owe us anything special. Our results are not perfect, nor are we. Rather, we have the rare privilege of doing something that we love, and simultaneously (most of the time) helping people. Once you believe you are infallible and have achieved the best results possible, you have failed as all learning has stopped.

Aspiring Towards Greatness

There are two things that separate a good plastic surgeon from a great plastic surgeon. One is the ability to properly evaluate the true underlying problem. The second is having the ability to develop innovative solutions to the problems. Being innovative means making minor or major adjustments to current techniques so that the procedure more specifically addresses the true underlying problems. This again reflects two of the three characteristics of a successful plastic surgeon: the power of observation and the gift of creativity and innovation.

Leadership in the Field

To be a true leader in most professions, you have to be an innovator. Plastic surgery is no different. You must be willing to think "out of the box" (i.e. rethink the "conventional wisdom"). Peers and patients alike respect someone who is putting forth that extra energy and effort to advance the field. A leader in the field of plastic surgery leads by example, by sharing knowledge, and by spending the time and energy to actively do whatever it takes to advance patient care and the plastic surgery profession.

Communicating with Patients

Communication is a key element in the level of patient's satisfaction as well as the third characteristic needed for success as a plastic surgeon. You can do the best job possible, but the patient will be dissatisfied if they were expecting something completely different because you did not communicate with them. In my practice, communication begins even before the patient comes in for their first visit. I have an extensive website that includes a number of the articles that I have written. These articles describe different techniques and state surgical goals, as well as reasonable expectations and recovery periods. The website has examples of possible results as shown through before and after pictures. Often before the patient comes in, my office mails them articles that I have written about the procedure in which they are interested.

When the patient comes for their first office visit, they usually meet with either my office nurse or the patient liaison office manager. This gives the patient an opportunity to sit with someone less initially intimidating than the "doctor" to discuss their basic medical history, areas of concern, and their motivations for surgery.

My staff then brings me "up-to-date" on the patient's issues and concerns so I can focus on their area of interest. Initially, I will ask follow-up questions that were not clear from the original interview with my staff. From then on, the patient and I evaluate their problem areas together. I take that opportunity to educate by explaining the reasons behind why the problem or deformity looks like it does, and what I feel is the proper way to approach each issue.

If during the communication process I feel their expectations are unreasonable or their motivations are not healthy, I will express my concerns. Once they understand my approach, I will discuss what is involved in performing the procedure, expected recovery, and potential risks with regard to specific procedures. During this first visit, patients spend about 1 1/2 - 2 hours in the office being educated. At the conclusion of the initial visit, I should have an informed patient with reasonable expectations regarding the proposed surgery.

The Most Difficult Part of "The Job"

I believe the most upsetting event for a plastic surgeon occurs when a patient is unhappy with the results of their procedure. For many of the best plastic surgeons this is the most difficult part of the profession. It is upsetting because much effort has gone into trying your best to be as creative and innovative as possible with the goal of making the patient happy.

How this disappointment is dealt with determines the ultimate outcome for patient and doctor. It is important to first step back and realize that the patient's criticisms are not personal. You then need to look at the situation objectively. Is the result a nice result, or is it a result that failed to meet obtainable goals? If it is a nice result and the person is not happy, then you need to remind the patient and yourself of the discussion about reasonable expectations that occurred prior to surgery. If it is a result that is not as satisfactory as the patient could have had, and they are justified in their concerns, we then discuss various options for improvement.

It is important for doctors and patients to realize that plastic surgeons cannot control everything that effects outcome. Sometimes the healing process does not go the way we expected. Many times, a postoperative complication requires supportive treatment, reassurance of the patient, and the promise that (if necessary) you will go back after the healing is complete and the inflammation is settled to try to improve what, if any, problems exist at that time.

Developing a Treatment Plan

In plastic surgery, the finer points involved in each procedure varies. As an example, let us examine how each facial rejuvenation procedure is different. Some people with aging faces have magnificent underlying bone structure and an adequate amount of facial fat. In those circumstances, you can reposition the fat on the facial bone structure and tighten the underlying muscles so that they look very attractive. Other people may have great bone structure, but their underlying facial fat has atrophied with age. In this instance, soft tissue augmentation (enhancement) with alloplastic (e.g. plastic or rubber) implants or autologous (a patient's own tissues such as fat or skin and fat together) implants will be required to achieve the best possible results. Marked asymmetry in the face will require adjustment of volumes and tissue tension from side to side. The key to understanding what is necessary in surgery is the understanding of what is wrong now. It is absolutely critical to have focused observation and a brutally honest evaluation in order to arrive at the true understanding of what should be done.

Attractive appearance post-surgery rarely comes by accident. Analysis of facial appearance can be mathematically quantified through facial proportions (the most important of which is the "Golden Ratio" as found in nature) and measured angles of facial projections. Body sculpting procedures are even more mathematical in planning and analysis. Just as a painter uses line drawings and measured sketches before the oil painting begins, the actual plastic surgery process of creation (or recreation) of beauty starts with mathematical analysis. Yet, in both cases, the process of artistic creation transcends the line drawings and mathematical guidelines with which one prepares. There is a traditional saying in plastic surgery: "measure twice, cut once" to which must be added "if the measurements don't appear to lend themselves to an aesthetically pleasing result, rethink the plan." The end product of surgery should be an attractive result, not pleasing numbers.

When No Plan is Satisfactory: Innovation

Sometimes there is no satisfactory answer to an aesthetic problem, or at least none has been described. An example of this occurred when confronting the problem of what to do with excess upper arm tissue and skin. Hanging arm tissue is a common problem that often bothers women who have gained and lost significant amounts of weight, or are genetically predisposed to have loose, large upper arms. The traditional way to treat this problem is to make an incision from the armpit down to the elbow. While this method is certainly direct, it usually results in a scar that no one wants. After thinking about this problem for years, I developed a new technique based on my experience with two seemingly unrelated procedures: liposuction of loose lower abdominal tissue and "purse string" type breast lifts. I had noted that after liposuction, the skin of even a hanging lower abdomen can shrink to flat. It is also well known that the wrinkled skin around the scar in a "purse string" type mastopexy almost always flattens and becomes smooth over several months. I hoped that by combining liposuction of the upper arm with a wide elliptical excision of axillary (armpit) skin, the following would happen: the upper arm tissues would be reduced in volume and shrink upward against the arm muscles, and the wrinkled scar in the armpit crease resulting from the loose skin excision would flatten and become barely perceptible. As a result, a successful procedure was invented to approach this problem. Now there is a very desirable alternative for the treatment of "batwing" arms compared to what was available only several years ago.

Scarring

It is oxymoronic on the surface to create beauty through creating scars, yet that dichotomy exists in my field. The elective scars are placed where they will have the best chance of healing into imperceptible lines. There are a number of things that can be done for patients to decrease the risk of unfavorable scarring. Initially, at the time of surgery, I close tissue in layers so that there is no tension on the outer skin. With no tension on the skin, the risk of having an unfavorable scar form is dramatically reduced.

Secondly, after the wound has healed for a couple of weeks, I like to use a yellow light pulse dye laser to treat the scar once or twice. In brief, the yellow light from the laser is absorbed by the capillaries in the skin. This process generates heat, causing a biochemical change to occur which in turn initiates a healing response. This healing response causes the skin and scar's collagen to become layered in organized sheets (similar to normal skin) as opposed to the tangles typical of scar tissue.

In addition, there are different topical ointments that can be put on scars to improve their character. These topical compounds range from silicone gel to onion extracts. More compounds are being discovered yearly.

Despite our best efforts, occasionally a bothersome scar develops. These more difficult scar problems may necessitate the injection of steroids alone or in combination with a chemotherapy drug (5-Flouro-uracil).

Keeping Up-to-Date with Technology

There are several ways of keeping up-to-date with all the new technological developments. You would think that reading the major plastic surgery journal articles would be the best way, but it is not. In general, most journal articles are about a year or more behind the most current concepts. If there is no other source of current information, then they can be very important. I find the best way for me to keep up-to-date is to constantly expose myself to new concepts and new ways of thinking about problems. This is why it is necessary to have a network of colleagues that you respect and with whom you can exchange ideas. The exchange of ideas and experiences with similar techniques allows a much more rapid building of new concepts and techniques than otherwise possible.

The technological advancements in the field of plastic surgery are much more difficult to fully appreciate. As a plastic surgeon, I am inundated with literature from companies and manufacturing representatives selling new technologies that they claim are the best. It is best to learn the truth about a purportedly wonderful, new technological advance by talking with someone who has used it. In the rare instances when a new technology arrives in the market, and the doctors I speak with have successfully used it, I will take a course in the technological advancement to learn more.

The Most Challenging Aspects of Being a Plastic Surgeon

Plastic surgery is an ever-changing and fascinating field. There lies its charm and challenge: excellence in the plastic surgery profession involves a constant learning process. Expertise yesterday does not confer expertise tomorrow. As with all experts driven to be the best in their field, the obstacles to continued expertise are multiple. The preceding discussion as to what is necessary to be one of the best plastic surgeons raises many of these obstacles for examination. Yet, these challenges would not be worth addressing if there were no reward.

The rewards for persevering and overcoming these obstacles to excellence are great. The rewards exceed the financial remuneration received. The rewards exceed the public commendations and the admiration expressed in the media for excellence in the field. The true reward of success is when, through hard work, planning and execution, a patient has a dramatic improvement in their quality of life. Dramatically improving another's life is a very precious reward few people experience on a regular basis. It is the ultimate reward we as humans can receive.

The Educational Highlights of a Plastic Surgeon

The training and lifelong commitment to learning involved in becoming a top plastic surgeon has been discussed above. Learning to be excellent entails developing wisdom. Wisdom entails observing and learning from what went right and what went wrong. Even failure, perhaps especially failure, is an opportunity to learn valuable lessons.

Honesty in self-evaluation and in perceiving the value of others' contributions is necessary for growth as an expert. The more interaction with excellence you are able to obtain, the larger the variety of ways you see available to approach problems. Consequently, this makes you better able to become an innovator in your field – the ultimate in creativity. When a plastic surgeon finishes the formal residency training, he will have a good basic education. However, it is not until one begins to "practice" the specialty that the real learning begins on how to evaluate, treat, approach, understand and conceptualize problems and their solutions.

Public Pitfalls in the Search for Aesthetic Plastic Surgery

There has been a significant increase over the past decade of non-board certified plastic surgeons who call themselves plastic surgeons in order to capitalize on the public's demand for aesthetic surgery. These unscrupulous individuals are attempting to perform procedures that should only be done by an experienced plastic surgeon. Their "training" in the field of plastic surgery could be as short as a weekend course. Their understanding and knowledge base in the field is miniscule. They put their patients at unacceptable risk.

These "pretenders" create a large public health issue. Obviously, patients are being misled, and are not getting the quality of care that they thought they would receive. Furthermore, this phenomenon is tarnishing the reputation of the real board certified plastic surgeons. This is a public health problem as well as a consumer fraud issue.

Positive Public Influences Regarding Plastic Surgery

On the positive side, the public demand for aesthetic surgery has been rapidly growing in response to seeing celebrities and shows like "Extreme Makeover." Despite plastic surgeons' initial anxiety about the "Extreme Makeover" show, it has been good for both the public and the profession, due to the integrity the show's producers have displayed in accurately representing the surgery, recovery, results, and ancillary issues that arise. They exclusively use board certified plastic surgeons to perform the plastic surgery. In many ways, this type of entertainment starts the educational process of making potential clients think about what is involved in their decision to proceed with aesthetic plastic surgery. It demonstrates how plastic surgery can change the way people feel about themselves, the way they project themselves and the way the interact in society. Yet, the show has been much more realistic than we thought it would be, and that has been good.

The Internet has been a fantastic influence on plastic surgery. Healthcare questions and research now exceed pornography as the highest use on the Internet. The Internet's availability to educate prospective plastic surgery patients prior to their visit makes a wonderful difference. A patient who has researched their plastic surgery topic of interest on the Internet and visited multiple sites, is much better educated. You can speak to this type of educated potential patient on a much higher level about procedures. Their level of understanding is deeper and their expectations more realistic.

Advances in the Field

There has been tremendous advancement over the past decade in biochemistry and laser biophysics. The topical applications with therapeutic creams and lasers allow us to treat patients more effectively with little if any recovery time. In the future, there will be further improvements in these topical treatments. Injectables will be further developed so that a well-tolerated injectable used to fill out wrinkles and inflate thinning areas will last significantly longer with less risk of reaction.

Another area of rapid advancement is in the area of breast implants. I have no doubt that in 15 years we will be looking back on the breast implants available today as antiquated devices. Yet, what we have now has been extensively researched and shown to be safe and effective.

Techniques evolve over time due to shared cumulative experience and those that always question: "How can the result be better?" From "Body Lifts" for those who had massive weight loss, to full facial rejuvenation of natural shape and appearance, the techniques I use have dramatically changed over the past 5 years alone.

Advice to a Young Plastic Surgeon

The first piece of advice I would tell every young plastic surgeon is to take care of each patient as you would a beloved family member. If you do not truly care about the result of the surgery for that patient, then you should not be their doctor. To deprive the patient and yourself of the empathy you should be feeling towards them, limits your ability to give the best you can, as well as prevents you from receiving the ultimate reward – the satisfaction of changing another's life for the better

Board certification in plastic surgery involves a long, but finite, training process. To become a successful plastic surgeon involves a lifetime commitment. Without that commitment you will do neither yourself nor your community a service. You need to evaluate whether this is a career that will bring you joy. Do you have a love of art, a tenacity of purpose, and the willingness to obtain the scientific knowledge necessary? Do you love this career above all others? Does the joy you receive from unleashing creativity exceed the pain you will feel from the sacrifices in your time, energy, and sleep? Are you able to accept the responsibility of caring for others, knowing that, despite your best efforts, failures occasionally occur? To be the best in any field requires hard work and dedication. To be the best in plastic surgery additionally requires a deep emotional commitment due to the sacrifices that will need to be made and the personal responsibility for others that you must assume.

Dr. Mark Richards is a recognized leader in cosmetic plastic surgery, as well as in the medical community. He has been interviewed by news columnists and television journalists alike for his expertise in plastic and laser surgery. Recent honors include selection by the Consumer's Research Council of America for inclusion in their Guide to America's Top Surgeons. Washingtonian Magazine selected Dr. Richards as one of the Washington D.C. metropolitan area's "top doctors." Baltimore Magazine lists Dr. Richards as "the doctor to go to" for body contouring and other plastic surgical procedures. He has received national acclaim for the surgery he performed on Linda Tripp. Patients travel across the US and from abroad to take advantage of his cosmetic surgery skills and expertise. In 1996 and 1998 Dr. Richards was honored nationally as being one of the Outstanding Young Men of America.

Dr. Richards graduated from Yale University with honors in 1979. He received his medical degree from the University of Maryland

School of Medicine in 1983. Dr. Richards then completed 5 years of residency training in general surgery, as well as an additional 2-year residency in plastic surgery. Dr. Richards has been certified by both the American Board of Surgery and the American Board of Plastic Surgery. In addition to his practice of 13 years, Dr. Richards has written on many topics in plastic surgery and lectured extensively to the medical and lay communities. The technique Dr. Richards developed to "lift" sagging arms with hidden incisions was published as the lead article in the July/August 2001 issue of the Aesthetic Surgery Journal. His article entitled "Patient Satisfaction After High-volume Lipoplasty: Outcomes Survey and Thoughts on Safety" was recently published in the Sept/Oct 2003 issue of the Aesthetic Surgery Journal.

Dr. Richards has served as President of the National Capitol Society of Plastic Surgeons (the MD, VA and Washington DC metropolitan area Plastic Surgery Society) and as President of the Montgomery County Medical Society (a 1700 member physician professional society dedicated to improving patient and community healthcare). Dr. Richards continues to update his skills and knowledge through many hours of continuing medical education (CME) and is a current member of the American Society of Plastic Surgeons (ASPS).

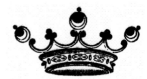

The ABCs of Plastic Surgery

Louis P. Bucky, M.D., FACS

Associate Professor of Surgery, Plastic Surgery
University of Pennsylvania School of Medicine

Basics of Plastic Surgery

The art of plastic surgery is to look at a defect or a problem, whether it's a wound-healing problem or an appearance problem, and visualize how the area can be reconstructed and improved. One has to be able to envision the ideal result and then determine how to create it. The other art of plastic surgery is understanding the needs of the patient. There is a patient need, both emotional and physical. Patients present varying body images. Understanding the impact of appearance on their personal, social and professional lives at the time of the consultation is critically important.

Plastic surgery requires the blending of art with science. The science of a plastic surgeon involves knowing how to keep tissue alive in addition to understanding the limitations of tissue viability. It is important to understand blood flow to determine how much viability of the tissue can be achieved. Sometimes it is necessary to use materials that are not living tissue, and a consummate knowledge of these materials is instrumental. Plastic surgery is really a combination of artistic visualization and a scientific understanding of tissues and non-living tissue materials in order to use those components to solve anatomic and functional deficits.

A plastic surgeon really needs to relate to patients and have empathy toward them and an understanding of how appearance-related problems affect their lives. It is important to appreciate how the patient perceives a problem in order to work with the patient to create a road map to solve it. The plastic surgeon must empathize with how bad a problem is for the patient. Sometimes a patient will see a relatively small flaw as a huge problem. It is important to take into account the patient's viewpoint and apply that to their treatment plan. If a patient has a small problem that is not consuming them, then the plastic surgeon will not perform a complex treatment that's going to involve a long recovery. On the other hand, if a patient is truly disabled by a condition and can't function well unless their wounds are healed or their breast is reconstructed, then sometimes a more sophisticated or complicated treatment plan may need to be offered.

Treating Patients

There are three important components in communicating with your patients. One is to listen well. The second is to present reasonable and realistic options. The third and perhaps most intriguing, particularly for the cosmetic patients, are visual tools such as computer imaging. Computer imaging provides a visual representation of the outcome of the procedure. Visual tools can provide a great deal of comfort in addition to a realistic depiction of the outcome. For example, if a patient is going to have a mastectomy and their abdomen will be used to make the new breast, they will most likely appreciate a visual aid in order to grasp this concept. If a patient comes in for a rhinoplasty or nasal surgery, computer imaging enables them to actually envision their appearance once they have completely healed. One of the interesting elements of plastic surgery is that while there are modifications from patient to patient, the underlying techniques are still founded on established operations and fundamentals. For instance, in breast reconstruction, if someone is missing skin and muscle from the chest, one tries to replace it with skin and muscle from a nearby area. For this reason, the abdomen's skin, muscle and fat are used to replace a breast, which is a structure comprised of skin and fat with underlying muscle.

In the cosmetic world, the strategy is to achieve the most natural result possible without causing any secondary deformities in addition to minimizing recovery. In cosmetic surgery, we tend to minimize any subsequent deformities because we are trying to enhance appearance as opposed to completely repairing missing tissue, which is what is done on the reconstructive side.

Technology

Plastic surgery is a field where there are always new developments. There are three main ways to keep current. One is to attend conferences and meetings – these are very helpful because experts in the field will present findings in panel discussions and abstracts. The second method is to keep up with the journals, which are timely and usually very well reviewed. The third option is to continually converse with a close group of colleagues in order to benefit from their experience in a more informal and interactive setting.

Future Advances

Modification of the treatment of scars would be a great advance. There is unpredictability about the way patients heal. Plastic surgery is a field where patients will trade scars or incisions for improvements in contour. They will choose a breast reduction, despite the fact that this surgery can result in significant incisions and scars, because they want a better shape. Or they will choose to have a tummy tuck, which requires an incision across the abdomen. There is a continual effort to generate new technology that would improve scarring and wound healing so patients would not have to make that trade-off.

There is a lot of room in plastic surgery to create and modify operations. The goal always is to try to find a simpler, less morbid treatment to improve the patient's result or solve their problem. With the advances in technology and the advances in our understanding of tissues, there are many ways to try to achieve those goals. In fact, there is a demand for development in plastic surgery almost unlike any other field.

There has been a big push toward less invasive procedures that allow patient improvements without the long recovery. In the cosmetic world, there are procedures for the skin that are non-surgical and that have had a big impact ranging from Botox® and fillers to laser treatments and skin care. These have really taken the lead over simply pulling the skin tighter. In the reconstructive world, there are devices that are healing wounds in a fashion that we were unable to do previously. These are two ends of the spectrum where technology has had a big impact.

Challenges of Being a Plastic Surgeon

One of the most difficult challenges of being a plastic surgeon is time management. Between surgery, office hours and research, family time and personal time is limited. Most plastic surgeons have the difficult task of balancing professional and personal time commitments.

Expectation management is another challenge. Today, people are bombarded by TV shows, newspapers and magazines that make plastic surgery seem simple and show patients and celebrities touched up to an ideal form. That is almost unachievable for most people. Therefore, spending the appropriate time to communicate to patients realistic expectations is important. Another challenge is that patients have the illusion that all patients just end up looking fabulous instantly, without a recovery, so getting them to understand that they will have a recovery period, and sometimes a long one, is another issue.

Sometimes it seems impossible to satisfy a patient's expectations. Whether it is a cosmetic or reconstructive patient, it can be very frustrating. It is important to keep in mind that this is human nature and people have their own issues. The good news is that it is very rare that a patient is unhappy with the ultimate result. If it happened a lot, this practice would be intolerable – there would be a constant feeling of failure.

What I personally dislike are the operations that are simply not successful. No matter how well a surgery is performed, there are risks, whether it's an infection or other complications. Complications can be very upsetting and difficult to accept. A good surgeon is one who manages his or her complications well and has the wherewithal to handle these issues and to effectively take care of patients.

The practice of medicine today is more challenging overall, with insurance-related issues and malpractice pressures, but those are secondary to being a plastic surgeon. Every physician in practice today has those problems.

Measuring Success

There are several ways to measure success. One is to set goals and to frequently monitor whether these goals are being achieved. Some goals stem from practice development -- thinking about the kinds of operations that the plastic surgeon prefers to do and what profile they would like their practice to have and then trying to get to that point. Another method is to quantitatively survey patients and ask them how the practice is doing in order to get feedback on whether patients are being served well. Last, at the end of the day nothing compares to the fulfillment that comes from having performed good surgery and having helped take care of patients. A good surgeon should expect to feel that way the vast majority of days.

Leadership

Leaders can be defined in many ways: there are leaders in teaching, leaders in development, leaders in political action, etc. It is important to have a clear vision as to what you want to accomplish. If you want to be the greatest teacher in plastic surgery, then that is your goal and you have to take the time to focus on that goal. Some leaders in plastic surgery are political activists who advocate for plastic surgery and its role in American medicine today. Some want to be involved in fixing the malpractice crisis. Others want to focus on surgical developments. Great leaders are those who can see what they want to achieve and where the problems are beyond what most people can and then have the personality and the tenacity to make it happen.

Finding the Right Doctor

The training that a board certified plastic surgeon goes through is the foundation. That involves learning from smart plastic surgeons who are dedicated teachers. Once you have that foundation, you can teach yourself a little bit about what works for you. Still, formal surgical training and continued education are the keys to a good practice of plastic surgery in the future.

The best way to select a plastic surgeon is to go by the ABCs. A is to ask people – other doctors, other patients – about a plastic surgeon. B is to check their background. There are people who claim to be board certified, but there is only one American Board of Medical Specialties (ABMS) Certification by the American Board of Plastic Surgery. Those who are certified by the ABMS have to undergo a certain amount of training and pass both written and oral examinations. The American Board of Plastic Surgery is the only plastic surgery field where people are truly ABMS certified. The C is consultation. It is in the consultation that the patient can either gain a comfort level that the surgeon will take good care of them or decide to further pursue their search.

Advice

Their is much to gain in trying to understand where the patient is coming from and then creating a surgical plan that will achieve those goals. In other words, a patient may come in with a problem that is minor to them and major to you; recommending too complex of an operation will likely cause strain. On the other hand, it may be that they think they have a big problem, but you think it's relatively insignificant and do not give it the appropriate emphasis. If you really listen, you can come up with a plan to help them.

The goals of being a good plastic surgeon should be first to establish a good relationship with your patients. You are a physician first and you need to understand the goals of the patient and how the problems can be treated. Second, lay out a clear surgical plan that has a good chance of being successful and, particularly, for the cosmetic patients, does no harm. You don't want to leave them worse off. Third, continue to care for your patents after the surgery and make sure that you have the ability to take care of any complications that occur. If these three objectives are accomplished, then you should have a successful outcome. The last and most important element is to only continue to practice if you love plastic surgery. If you find that you don't love it anymore, it's time to find another career.

Louis P. Bucky, M.D., FACS, is an Associate Professor of Surgery within the Division of Plastic Surgery at the U. of Pennsylvania School of Medicine. Dr. Bucky received his medical degree from Harvard Medical School. He trained at the Massachusetts General Hospital in Boston, MA, the Memorial Sloane-Kettering Cancer

Center in New York and Miami Children's Hospital. Dr. Bucky is board certified in General Surgery and Plastic Surgery. He is a member of several regional and national societies, including the American Society of Plastic Surgery, the American Society of Aesthetic Surgery, and the Northeastern Plastic Surgery Society. He is a fellow of the American College of Surgeons.

His clinical work has been featured in Plastic Surgery Journals, MAMM Magazine, Family Circle, Redbook, Good Morning America, and CNN. Recently, Dr. Bucky was named a "TOP DOC" in Philadelphia Magazine and included in the prestigious "America's Top Doctors."

Dr. Bucky practices at Pennsylvania Hospital, the Hospital of the University of Pennsylvania, and the Children's Hospital of Philadelphia. He holds appointments at the University of Pennsylvania Cancer Center, The Rena Rowan Breast Cancer Center and the Pigmented Lesion Group.

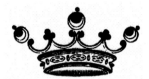

Communicating with the Patient

Michael Olding, M.D., FACS

Chief, Division of Plastic and Reconstructive Surgery & Associate Professor of Surgery, George Washington University Medical Center; *Director,* Cosmetic Surgery and Laser Center

The Artistry of Plastic Surgery

Plastic surgery is part art, part science. Although the science of plastic surgery can be taught, artistic appreciation for and execution of techniques which enhance beauty are more subjective and therefore more difficult to teach. Plastic surgeons should possess some innate talent and sense of artistry, as well as the desire to utilize techniques designed to fully express that artistic sense. Mastered under the tutelage of those more experienced during a rigorous training program, the end product is a plastic surgeon that can draw upon various learned techniques to accomplish an aesthetic result, which must be both pleasing and natural. The term plastic surgery comes from the word "plastikos," which means fit for molding. We have the ability to reshape the face and body, but must remember that "different" is not necessarily "better." It is in part that artistic sense at play, which is so important to the successful plastic surgeon. Unfortunately we have all seen examples of plastic surgery gone awry – breasts which have been over enhanced, faces which have been pulled too tight and mask-like, and noses which have been carved away leaving only a remnant of what previously existed.

There is an acceptable standard of beauty, which is different in different societies. The average person may not be able to articulate what that standard is, but everyone recognizes when someone falls far outside that acceptable standard. Today, patients are looking for more natural results, and we have a responsibility to deliver them. Can the patient have a great result and still be unhappy? Of course they can, unless time is spent with the patient to discuss the subtle aspects of the surgery and the tradeoffs which might occur.

The good plastic surgeon needs to be part artist, sculptor, hand holder, and cheerleader. Although plastic surgery requires an understanding of science and new technologies, it also requires a more thorough understanding of patients than is required for other types of surgery. For example, if a patient requires an appendectomy, there is no discussion of the past psychological history or the many other life experiences – if the surgery is performed in a skilled fashion, removing the appendix, then the surgery is a success. Not so with plastic surgery. Only when many variables and subjective evaluations of the result as well as the skillful completion of the surgery are taken into consideration, can the final result be deemed successful. Although we operate on the face and body, those operations have profound effects on the psychological well being and confidence of the patient. Therefore, a good rapport between the surgeon and patient is essential to a "good" result.

Establishing a Good Doctor-Patient Relationship

More than anything else, plastic surgeons are patient advocates. The doctor-patient relationship is a two-way street. There must be an exchange of dialogue between the two rather than from one (the doctor) to the other (the patient). It is unlike many other types of doctor-patient relationships in that the decision about what to do and how much to do is dependent upon that interaction, usually during the first consultation. I do not consider it my role to "tell" the patient that they need procedure X, procedure Y, or procedure Z. Rather, we together come to a decision about what I can accomplish surgically, and what will improve their aesthetic result. Concern, compassion and honesty are critical components of this dialogue, not hype, glitz, and self-promotion. Today's reality TV shows over-glamorize the plastic surgeon, and do much to undermine our perceived integrity. Hollywood is not necessarily reality, and cosmetic surgery is no longer only available to the idle rich. Modern day prospective cosmetic surgery patients are more educated than ever before about the different alternatives available and in many ways this makes my job easier. Dialogue becomes more meaningful and instructive if the patient has done suitable background work regarding the surgery.

Ideally, communication with patients involves sitting down with them in a comfortable environment, spending any amount of time needed to answer their questions, and fully educating them about what they are considering so that there are no misunderstandings about the risks and benefits of a procedure. But realistically, you can't always be certain that a patient completely understands the procedure. Usually before a patient arrives at a plastic surgeon's office, he or she has been sent informational brochures about the procedure being considered or they have researched the cosmetic surgery on the Internet. It's a great source of information both about the surgery and about the surgeon. In fact, we often receive referrals from the Internet or magazines that rank the best plastic surgeons. Patients have an idea of not only what they want but also whom they want because they've already done some shopping around.

When Plastic Surgery is the Right Choice

There are no age restrictions on reconstructive surgery. Because some things require immediate attention, such as the case of a newborn with cleft lip and palate, a plastic surgeon must take into account special situations and circumstances and assess each patient's needs on a case-by-case basis. For example, I do not routinely perform cosmetic surgery on teenagers, but there are exceptions to that rule. The most commonly discussed issue among young girls is breast augmentation. In my opinion, this procedure is inappropriate for teenagers. I have, however, performed augmentation when there has been a congenital deformity and there is almost no breast or muscle on one side, and a normal breast on the other. I do not consider that a cosmetic procedure, although it is an augmentation on one side.

Whereas, many teenagers undergo cosmetic rhinoplasty (nose job) and otoplasty (ear pinning) without any concern, breast augmentation in young women must be viewed with great speculation.

No plastic surgeon, no physician, can do everything well. If I am uncertain what to do in a particular case, I seek opinions from other people. If a patient is looking for a type of surgery with which I have limited experience, I will refer that patient to a doctor who specializes in that area. You cannot perform an operation once every other year and expect to get a good result for your patient. I advocate second opinions whenever the patient (or doctor) is not 100 percent convinced about the suitability of the operation.

One of the most challenging aspects of being a plastic surgeon is knowing who is a good candidate for a procedure and who will be happy with what can be delivered. Even though *you* deliver what you consider a good result, you cannot be certain that the *patient* will consider it a good result. What is considered a positive outcome is very subjective.

If a patient is unhappy with the results of the surgery, I try to determine the cause of the dissatisfaction. There could be a complication that may or may not be reversible, depending on the nature of the problem. You assess the situation and address it – as well as possible solutions – with the patient. You need to determine if it is something that can be treated with additional surgery. For example, if you have a face-lift, there are many, many factors that can determine whether or not you get the perfect result. Early in the postoperative process, noticeable lumps and scarring can appear. These are expected in the early postoperative period. Because there are many changes, which occur during the first months after the surgery, I nearly always wait a full year before performing any revisional surgery on a patient because during that time, many of the minor scars, lumps and bumps will disappear.

The more educated patients are, the more prepared, and the more real are their expectations. I want them to understand that, as with any surgery, the potential for complications exists. Even though the risks may be minimal, the informed consent that patients must sign discusses possible complications. Videotapes are also helpful in explaining the possible benefits and complications of a procedure.

It is important for plastic surgeons to address psychological issues directly. Discussing any history of mental illness or depression, as well as pertinent medications, is essential if you are looking to do what is best for the patient. It is not a good idea for patients who are unhappy or depressed or have a mental illness to turn to plastic surgery as a way to solve their problems. Those types of problems are often deep-seeded, not situational, and often only masked or worsened by the surgery. The most ideal time to consider cosmetic surgery is when the patient is the happiest.

Two types of cases come up most frequently in relation to psychological issues. One is if there is a long-term psychiatric problem, such as long-term depression. If someone has a history of mental illness, it does not necessarily mean that they shouldn't have cosmetic surgery. But this type of patient needs to understand that the surgery isn't going to cure his or her depression. The second type of patient is one who is reacting to a situational problem. For example, an individual who has been left by a spouse after many years of marriage may seek plastic surgery as a reaction to situational depression. In my opinion, these types of patients are not good candidates for cosmetic surgery at that moment in time. It would be best if they wait until they are in a better frame of mind before they make a surgical decision.

Success as a Surgeon

There are several factors that contribute to a plastic surgeon being successful. First, you need to enjoy what you're doing. If you do not like what you are doing, you are not going to do your best. Second, you need to have some innate abilities such as manual dexterity and an artistic sense. Third, you have to be meticulous to a fault. If you are not, the final results may be acceptable but they may not be great, and great is what patients want. When people look in the mirror each day, they are going to expect a result that improves their sense of well being and their quality of life.

The best way to learn the skills of successful plastic surgery is to complete a plastic surgery residency. These training programs have very specific educational objectives. To become board-certified in plastic surgery, residents must successfully complete the program and then take a special test in order to be board-certified by the American Board of Plastic Surgery.

It is important for plastic surgeons to be innovative and to try new things as long as safety remains a priority. The risk of trying a new technique is that there are no results available from long-term testing that can help you assess the positives and negatives. Silicone injections are a good example. When the injections were being administered on a regular basis 30 or 40 years ago, everyone thought they were great. They were seen as a safe, easy, and effective means of filling in lines. But after 15 or 20 years, patients started experiencing problems with granuloma formation. Today, injections of silicone in soft tissues, is not approved in the United States. When silicone injections first came on the market they seemed innovative, but it turns out that they were not safe. It is important to thoroughly evaluate and research new techniques before you perform them.

You base your success as a surgeon on several things – what your patients say, how your fellow physicians regard your work, your reputation in the community, your recognition in a more national forum. But more than anything else, you base how successfully you have performed a procedure on feedback from your patients. To become a leader – whether in plastic surgery or in any other field – you need motivation that goes beyond any financial concerns. You need to have the drive to continually learn, improve, and judge your results with a critical eye.

What the Future Looks Like

The principles of plastic surgery have not changed much in recent years. What has changed is the amount of information available to the public about plastic surgery and the media promotion of cosmetic procedures. This type of surgery has become much more acceptable and commonplace, and also more affordable. There have been many advances in technology, which means we can offer patients many more treatment alternatives. There are many continuing medical educational programs available to hone new techniques and learn about pitfalls that others may have experienced in using a particular technique.

Today's patients are opting for less invasive procedures at an earlier age. Non-surgical alternatives are particularly attractive to patients, especially ones that have little down time from work (and play). Botox has almost been a national phenomenon. It paralyses facial muscles therefore decreases unwanted lines. In the immediate future we will see significant increases in the number of "fillers." In addition to collagen, many new fillers will be available to fill out the lines in the face as well as to restore the fullness in areas where aging or scars have left a deficiency. Many of the new products coming out will make a tremendous difference in the entire field of cosmetic surgery. Five or ten years ago laser treatments made big headlines; now it is going to be fillers. There will be fillers which no longer require a skin test, so that more people are candidates for the procedure. The other products either available or soon to be available are made from hylaruonic acid, calcium hydroxylapatite, human-based collagen implant, and microshperes of PMMA, which last many years. There have also been great advances made in the injection of ones own fat, so that now techniques result in permanent improvement with fat injection alone.

There will be more impetus to find a better breast implant. The FDA will be heavily involved in approving any new implants that are brought to market, but the approval process for this type of product doesn't happen overnight. Implants are much better than they were ten years ago, and they will be better ten years from now. Although there was a great deal of controversy over silicone gel implants, the bulk of the medical science has found them safe. There has been no link with systemic disease.

I think that plastic surgery will always be one of the most interesting surgical specialties. Every procedure is an opportunity to impact someone's life and help him or her realize a goal. It is important to recognize that every patient is an individual with his or her own expectations. As plastic surgeons, we can offer guidance, opinions, and ultimately, our expertise to bring about a positive change. Cosmetic surgery is far from frivolous. Both plastic surgeons and patients should always remember that its effects, most often, are long lasting. But plastic surgery alone can never be expected to change all aspects of an individual's life.

Dr. Olding is Chief of Plastic Surgery at The George Washington University Medical Center and director of the Cosmetic Surgery and Laser Center. He is board certified by the American Board of Plastic Surgery. He is a Fellow of the American College of Surgeons, and a member of the American Society of Plastic Surgeons. He has received numerous awards and fellowships for his work and has lectured internationally. He maintains a busy cosmetic surgery practice in Washington D.C.

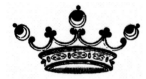

Envisioning the End Result

David T.W. Chiu, M.D., FACS, FAAP

Director, New York Nerve Center &
Clinical Professor of Surgery
New York University Medical Center

The Artistry of Plastic Surgery

In his eloquent forward to the treatise of Gillies and Millard, *The Principles and Art of Plastic Surgery*, the late Dr. Jerome P. Webster quoted the words of Aristotle, as it appeared in his work *On the Parts of Animals*: "Art, indeed, consists in the conception of the result to be produced before its realization in the material." He then elaborated, "An artist, therefore, must not only be able to conceive the end result to be produced, but he must also be able to visualize all the necessary steps leading to that end, and he must have the imagination, the intelligence, and the dexterity to bring about that result. Is not, then, plastic surgery an art, and the plastic surgeon an artist?"

In essence, a plastic surgeon, like an artist, must have the faculty to conceptualize and visualize an end result, and further more, the capability to configure the road to reach that result.

In addition to artistry, plastic surgery has an equally important scientific dimension. A plastic surgeon must be attuned with the physiology of wound healing, the anatomy of vasculature, and biochemistry and cellular biology of immunorejection phenomena. A plastic surgeon is often charged with the duty to moderate the effects arising from the interplay of the art and science of surgery for their patients.

One way to gain a better insight of plastic surgery is to study what a plastic surgeon does. Using my own experience of more than two decades as an example, where I have been privileged to have been called upon to solve a rather diverse group of problems, I can classify my work into the following categories: 1) Refinement: 2) Resection: 3) Repairment; 4) Replantation; 5) Reconstruction.

To *refine* is to add when there is overt deficiency and to reduce when there is burdensome excess. The respective remedy for the aforementioned problems, namely, augmentation mammoplasty and reduction mammoplasty, are two good contrasting examples. These types of procedures fall into the group known as cosmetic surgery. Another common cosmetic operation is rhytidectomy, also know as a facelift. This type of operation is to minimize the wrinkles of the skin and to restore the youthful linearity of the facial feature in order to narrow the gap between how the patient thinks they should look and what they actually see in the mirror. If the patient's expectation is realistic, he or she will often benefit from such a surgical endeavor.

To *resect* is to remove aberrant structure causing compression of other vital structure(s), or to remove a tumorous growth. Resection of the transverse carpal ligament, as in Carpal Tunnel Syndrome, and parotidectomy for extirpation of a tumor of the parotid gland with preservation of the facial nerves, are common examples.

To *repair* is to restore the integrity of injured structures which were normal prior to a physical insult, often as a result of trauma. For example, repair of lacerated tendons, nerves, vessels, bones, and skin resulting from snow blower accidents are sadly frequent in the winter days.

To *replant* is to reattach a severed body part. Advent of microsurgery over the last three decades rendered anastomosis of vessels as small as 0.5 mm in diameter with over a 90 percent success rate, giving many of our patients a second chance to regain use of lost body parts, such as fingers, hands, arms, legs, ears and male genitalia.

To *reconstruct* is to replace structures that are missing as a result of congenital anomaly, trauma, or disease. The goal is to restore missing functions and structures toward normalcy. Here the principles of reduction through prioritization and reconstruction through redistribution apply. When a baby is born with no thumb and only two fingers, as one finds in the case of amniotic band syndrome, I have utilized microsurgery to transfer a vascularized second toe from each foot to build a thumb and an additional finger to restore a cascade of a four digit hand.

Challenges and Creativity

Plastic surgeons are trained to be problem solvers, and are expected to be creative in coming up with solutions whenever presented with challenging situations. In fact many of us are attracted to plastic surgery because it is a field wherein creativity can flourish. In addition, many plastic surgeons by nature are perfectionists. Some, by training, become perfectionists. As a group, we have the proclivity to take on new task with gusto, and strive to achieve perfect results with passion. The progress we have made, and the high standards we have set in microsurgery over the last three decades, are vivid examples of the formidable combination of these traits. Yet, when we are happily and eagerly exercising our creativity and striving for perfection, we must remain vigilant to our human limitations.

Presenting a creative solution to a patient requires setting realistic goals accurately, reflective of our ability and moderated by wisdom of humility. If we present ourselves as a superhero, we can set the patient's expectations too high, and a successful procedure may turn out to be a serious disappointment. Moderation in how we approach our work is beneficial to us and to our patients. It is important that we strike a balance between being a perfectionist and being a human – between being innovative and being realistic. This is a delicate balance that we must address constantly.

Communicating With Patients

Direct communication is usually the best method for conveying to a patient what a procedure involves and what they can expect. There are times when I draw out the procedure on paper, explaining the specifics to the patient as I go along. I go through the procedure, step by step, just to be sure that my patients understand the plan and have an idea of what to expect from the proposed treatment plan. I find this means of communication much more effective than throwing out Greek or Latin terms that don't clearly convey what an operation truly involves.

Cosmetic surgery patients, more so than reconstructive surgery patients, require more in-depth consultation with regards to their psychological profile. I would advise against cosmetic surgery in patients recently emerging from emotional upheaval. I believe that patients should make this kind of decision with the calmest of mind.

With cosmetic surgery patients, I begin by inquiring the reason for their visit. I would like them to point out to me the specific areas of their concern. If the area of complaint is physically identifiable and their expected degree of improvement is realistically achievable, I will then further our discussion to various alternative approaches.

Most people are very, very specific about their desires. The plastic surgeon must then review all of the benefits, risks, and alternatives involved in meeting a desired goal. In terms of risks, I generally discuss the common risks of every surgery as well as the specific risks of plastic surgery. For example, with rhinoplasty you need to decide whether to perform an open or closed rhinoplasty. A closed rhinoplasty involves making an incision inside the nose so you don't see the scar. An open rhinoplasty involves opening up the skin, creating an incision, and peeling back the skin to examine the cartilage and bone; in this way, you can do much more precise sculpturing or replacement. Opening up the skin brings added risks but also added benefits. The plastic surgeon needs to guide the patient toward the most sensible choice. Much of the decision rests with patient and his or her ability to tolerate risk. It is not a matter of the surgeon dictating what the patient should do.

A plastic surgeon is responsible for telling the patient the likely outcome of the procedure. At the end of the discussion the patient and surgeon should be in agreement on how to proceed. Personally, I often want to feel that the patient and I are working together as a team. A patient's cooperation is critical to the success of a surgery. Likewise, the patient has to feel confidence in the surgeon and the procedure being proposed. Rapport between doctor and patient must be established before you proceed to the next steps of exploring when, how, and where to perform the operation.

Every surgeon handles his or her consultations differently. After the initial consultation, I suggest to patients that they take some time to digest all the information that has been conveyed, and to share that with their family. If a patient decides to pursue the operation, I insist the patient come back for a second consultation. For those who are married, I insist on meeting with their spouse. I would not operate on any married person without the unequivocal support of their spouse.

Roadblocks to Effective Treatment

In general, if you spend a sufficient amount of time analyzing and preparing for each case, you lessen the likelihood of encountering obstacles or roadblocks that hinder the success of a surgery. When a procedure does not go according to plan, you should step back and reassess the diagnosis you made and the information that was available to you. There are situations when additional data derives from additional testing, such as a biopsy with frozen section study. Such is the case when one unexpectedly finds a small but hard mass when performing a reduction mammoplasty. If the roadblock is not resolvable, abort the operation to gain a chance to re-evaluate, research, and revise the formulation of treatment. Never allow yourself to descend from uncertainty to desperation.

The Successful Plastic Surgeon

Becoming a successful plastic surgeon requires the same skills needed to be a good physician of any kind. First and foremost, you need to be a good listener. You must be able to empathize with a patient's desires and needs - both spoken and unspoken. You must be an astute diagnostician, and a skilled problem solver. You must be clear in your sense of priority. When available donor motor units are limited, rebuild the most essential, functional part first. Learn to compromise in order to simplify. Discipline yourself to reduce a long, seemingly impossible laundry list into an achievable formulation – thus the principle of progression through reduction. Cultivate the ability to communicate your suggestions and solutions in a manner that the patient can understand. Drawing out the procedure on a piece of paper can be very useful to help your patient visualize the operation and gain confidence in you. Always have back-up plans. When you have a whole set of possible scenarios laid out and alternative solutions all formulated, you often don't need to use them, since the beneficial consequence of a critical analysis and deduction is a well chosen course of action and a successful outcome.

While it is essential to be sharp as a diagnostician, thorough as a strategist, and methodical as an architect, you also have to be very commanding as a conductor, and very facile as a virtuoso. One essential faculty in operating surgery, seldom mentioned, is gentleness in tissue handling, which contributes greatly to minimize tissue trauma and thus postoperative discomfort.

Personally, I measure success by the level of satisfaction that my patients feel. The smile on a patient's face is my biggest joy. I feel a great sense of accomplishment when I analyze what I have done, look at the results, and realize that I have made a positive and significant difference in a patient's life. There is great satisfaction in helping people to feel better and to feel more energized and capable. When the surgery I have performed enables a patient to pick up a fork and eat independently again, or drive again, or feel a child's face again – that is when I feel that I have achieved something meaningful. To me, that is success.

Strategies for Learning Plastic Surgery

Plastic surgery is a very inclusive specialty. It interphases with practically every domain in medicine, ranging from dermatology to psychiatry. The sheer amount of pertinent information continuously being generated can be overwhelming. My strategy for managing the new information is like that of decorating a Christmas tree. Each branch represents a specific discipline. Within each discipline, I further subdivide them in accordance to organ system. These constitute the trunk, the corpus of my memory tree. Each piece of new information will be neatly placed on a special twig. There will be no loose angels floating around.

The strategy I use when I come up with a new technique is to develop an animal model to practice on. When I develop a new operation, I work out the fine details on fresh cadaver dissection.

A Look at the Changes in Plastic Surgery

During the last two decades, microsurgery has brought about dramatic changes in the world of plastic surgery. Today, we see a surge of interest in nerve regeneration and how nerves can be repaired. We have learned that you can repair nerves with the help of a microscope, and that you can get wonderful results. We also now know that if a nerve is missing a segment, you can borrow a segment of nerve from another area of the body. You can use the borrowed segment as a bridge to fill the gap.

One of the techniques that I was fortunate to discover is the use of a vein segment to bridge the gap of a nerve. The use of a segment of vein harvested from the same person provides a vital passage protected from scar tissue invasion yet physiologically amicable for the regenerating axons to traverse from the proximal stump to the distal stump unhindered. This technique is not only useful as a means for repairing a nerve with a gap, but also helpful in providing a window for the study of the mystery of nerve regeneration. By analyzing what type of cell is emerged in that tube, and in what order and time frame, we can learn much more about nerve regeneration. We now need to look further and analyze what kind of molecule emerges from that tube. Analyzing the molecule and its effect on nerve regeneration might enable us to impact the regeneration process. This would be a wonderful breakthrough in terms of treating nerve injuries. All of this new information about nerve regeneration is one of the most exciting medical developments in the last decade.

In the coming decade there may be tremendous changes in the area of molecular biology. New discoveries could affect the natural process of healing or aging. For instance, we have wrinkles because we lose skin elasticity; if we find a way to replenish the elasticity then we may not need face lifts.

Keeping Current

Reading medical journals is an excellent way to keep up with new developments and technologies. Another way to stay on top of trends and keep abreast with new development is to attend specialty society annual meetings. Yet the most effective way to keep current is to engage in research. When you are actively involved in research you not only peregrinate in the forefront of that realm of knowledge, but also contribute to expanding the horizon of plastic surgery.

It is critically important to be innovative in plastic surgery. Oftentimes a plastic surgeon comes up with a new idea, perfects the technique, and then everyone else starts using it. For example, skin grafting was perfected by one plastic surgeon; it is now widely practiced. During the last two decades microsurgery techniques were perfected primarily by plastic surgeons. Instead of moving the skin flap from one place to another, today we can take the flap, dissect out the artery and veins, and relocate them. Microsurgery is one of the many areas in which plastic surgery has continued to develop and grow. During the1920s and 30s we perfected skin grafting; during the 1970s and 80s we revolutionized microsurgery. The next 20 years could bring equally dramatic changes. As long as we continue to commit time and resources to finding better techniques, and as long as we continue to think creatively, I am certain plastic surgery will continue to be an innovative medical specialty.

Finding Satisfaction in Plastic Surgery

I often tell students that plastic surgery, being a functionally defined specialty, is not limited by any organ system boundary. In plastic surgery you are only limited by your imagination. You need to enjoy the challenge of the unknown. There is no cookbook for plastic surgery.

In terms of surgical remuneration, there are significant inequities in plastic surgery. If you devote your life to performing microsurgical reconstruction on patients with Medicare insurance, most likely you will not be able to sustain a viable practice, since the Medicare reimbursement for microsurgical operation is way below the overhead level. I believe that diversification is the sensible route to take. You should be open to embarking on any type of surgical undertaking as long as you have a genuine interest and maintain a high level of competency in it. If you want to do challenging work and at the same time remain solvent, my advice is to consider diversifying and maintaining a balanced practice. This is a very practical way of dealing with economic realities while doing the work that you love.

To succeed as a plastic surgeon you have to have a true passion for this field, and have a dedication that is genuine and long lasting. We have opportunities to make real change in patients' lives -- we refine, we repair, we replant, we resect, and we reconstruct. In plastic surgery you are given almost endless opportunities and the freedom to test the limits of both your imagination and your resolve to stretch the horizon.

David T.W. Chiu, M.D., F.A.C.S., F.A.A.P, obtained his M.D. from Columbia University. He is on the faculty at Columbia University and New York University's School of Medicine. He is a member of the finance committee at St. Mary's Hospital and a member of the International Editorial Board and the Journal of Reconstructive Microsurgery. Dr. Chiu is the Director of the New York Nerve

Center at *NYU Medical Center. He has received numerous awards for outstanding achievement in his field.*

Dedication *– This chapter is dedicated to the memory of the late Dr. Jerome P. Webster. It is through his patient and enlightening tutorage that I acquired the appreciation of plastic surgery as an art , and began my learning of plastic surgery as a science.*

Acknowledgement *– I would like to acknowledge the contribution of Laura Kearns in the writing of this chapter which is based on a stimulating interview that she thoughtfully orchestrated.*

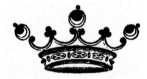

The Evolution of Plastic Surgery

Amitabha Mitra, M.D., FACS

Professor and Chief of Plastic Surgery
Temple University Health Sciences Center

Plastic Surgery vs. General Surgery

Plastic surgery, to a great extent, is entirely different from other surgical specialties. A plastic surgeon is essentially faced with challenging situations for which there are no specific and singular answers.

With appendicitis, you know the routine of the treatment plan. The patient takes antibiotics for a few hours, receives an IV, and then undergoes an operation. We cannot even dream of performing plastic surgery the same way we did 30 years ago. The same is not true about appendectomies. We do them exactly the same way today as we did 30 years ago, maybe with a different approach. Plastic surgery is a far more dynamic specialty.

The discipline of plastic surgery encompasses a wide variety of surgeries. We can essentially restore whatever is damaged from head to toe. Injuries to the face, like a broken jawbone or eye bone, may call for plastic surgery. If you break your skull and have an injury to the brain, you go to the neurosurgeon. But after the neurosurgeon has done the operation, there may be a defect in the skull that is visible from outside. The plastic surgeon is called in to fill in the defect and make it look as if there never was a defect.

Burn cases are another example. A plastic surgeon is a specialist who is expert in the management of cuts in the body, injuries to the hand and other extremities where bone, tendons and nerves exist. They work with orthopedics and other specialists. Plastic surgeons are called in to reattach amputated limbs and digits. When an individual sustains an open wound with a broken bone, a plastic surgeon is called in to cover the wound or bridge the bone. He or she is also the specialist who helps the orthopedists to heal a non-healing fracture by covering the affected bone with flaps which brings new blood supply to the area.

The evolution of the field of plastic surgery is like a Banyan tree, which is a huge Asian tree. A Banyan tree grows from a main trunk like any other tree. But the unique feature of this tree is that from its branches roots grow and descend into the ground and new roots and a trunk grow which in turn gives rise to another tree and the process continues. In this way the main tree and subsequent offspring grow wider and spread to cover a large area. Thus, just like a Banyan tree, plastic surgery has evolved from reconstruction to correction of congenital defects like cleft lip and palate, craniofacial defects, burn reconstruction, bone and hand surgery, microvascular surgery, post cancer reconstruction, etc. The experience of reconstruction has led us to the outcome of aesthetics. This in turn has evolved into the practice of cosmetic surgery. Modern day plastic surgery started with people who were injured in World War II, and it has now expanded to all kinds of reconstruction from head to toe.

Reconstructive and Aesthetic Aspects

In the progression from reconstructive to aesthetic, there is first, for example, breast cancer, which may lead to a mastectomy, or removal of breast tissue, which the woman may desire to have reconstructed, or restored to a natural-looking state.

Surgeons decided that if they could do that, it may be possible to make a small breast bigger, or make a big breast smaller. Then the focus became the nose, then the face. Nose reconstruction, or rhinoplasty, breast augmentation, and tummy tucks all began to some extent as reconstructive processes, branching later into aesthetics.

Plastic surgeon is limited by the imagination. We have the basic thought processes for how to correct things from head to toe. We can often apply the same principles of what we do for the head to what we do for the toe. For instance, we know how to take a toe out, so why can't we reconstruct the toe into a thumb so we could do what we call a toe-to-thumb transfer.

The Role of the Surgeon

There are two kinds of plastic surgeons. One type is reconstructive in character. The surgeon's compassion allows him to stay committed to a patient's defect or deformity, whether it is congenital or acquired from a disease or injury. An example would be a burn, which can be a very horrifying injury, and the surgeon treating such a case should be able to stay on the case for as long as it takes to keep that person alive and to make the patient look good, even if it takes six or seven operations or kinds of treatment.

The second group of plastic surgeons is more interested in the improvement of patients' body image. Individuals may feel as though they can't live their lives looking as they do, even if they have no defect. A plastic surgeon must be understanding, and not judgmental, as they make decisions about what should be done to improve these individuals' appearance and their perception of their own body image and make them feel functional in society and comfortable amongst their friends and colleagues. Present society sometimes can be unforgiving about the appearance of these individuals.

Qualities and Skills

Plastic surgeons must be well trained, of course, have technical skills, and be a broad-based general surgeon. They should know how to cut, stitch, and be very precise. A plastic surgeon has to have finesse and be a perfectionist.

A good plastic surgeon is three-dimensional. They also must have an imaginative capability and a broad understanding of the human body, as well as the human mind.

The human mind becomes important because the surgeon must understand which patients are acceptable candidates for having plastic surgery and which patients may not be reasonable when it comes to surgery. Understanding the patient and his or her realistic expectation of the outcome could be the difference between success and failure in surgery.

Communication with Patients

Communicating with plastic surgery patients is no different from communicating as a general physician. A good listener of the patient makes a good physician. A good history taker of patient ailment usually makes a good diagnosis and thus avoids wrong treatment. You listen to them to find out what level of understanding the person has. If you are a good doctor, you should be able to communicate at the level of the patient. Avoid talking down to them.

A doubtful patient is actually a better patient. A patient who has doubts is not sure. And if he is not sure, then it is the doctor's responsibility to explain things to him. Even the most illiterate individual or the greatest derelict in the streets can be helped to understand. You can explain to them the problems and the solutions. A knowledgeable physician is capable of explaining most of the medical problem to any patient without resorting to big words and medical jargons. Overall, patients with more questions are better patients.

Diagnosing the Problem

The training for diagnosing and treating patients is the same for all medical fields. Diagnosing a medical problem is the skill you learn in medical school and during your general residency. One has to have knowledge of differential diagnosis and a management plan based on proper investigative tools. A comprehensive history taking skill combined with use of proper investigations usually leads to correct diagnosis. Solid clinical knowledge also avoids use of unnecessary and sometimes costly investigations. In Hindu prayer ceremony the priest throws rice in the fire in the name of a specific god. Each time he throws rice, he or she watches intently to see if it catches fire. The rice with the name of the specific god which does not catch fire is eliminated from prayer. The one which does will call for elaborate prayer for that specific god as it is believed that the specific god is present in that time in that prayer center. Differential diagnosis at its basic form. A physician confronted with a diagnostic problem also throws a number of possible diagnoses in the pot. Patients' history and clinical findings eliminate certain diagnoses and hopefully he or she is left with few questions. The physician then uses the diagnostic tools like laboratory work up, X rays, Cat scans, etc., to come to a reasonable conclusion about possible problems. He or she may have a variety of treatment options. He or she chooses the right one for the patient. Because of my training and experience, the array of differential diagnosis and solutions come rather quick. But the process of thinking through remains the same. Patients ultimately help one to make the right decision.

I receive photographs sent to me from all over the world. Occasionally I have to say I don't recognize the problem. But when I show the photo around, someone eventually will say he has seen a similar kind of problem. After doing more research, we can send back information we have tracked. Being at the University I have the advantage of availability of world renowned experts at hand to bounce questions off.

Immediate and Delayed Complications

No surgical procedure should be taken lightly. Complications of surgery are totally unpredictable. Our goal is to identify the possible risks and prevent them as much as possible. A knowledgeable patient is a surgeon's best friend. There are certain things patients can do to avoid complications like cessation of smoking or following the medical directions given to the patient both pre- and post-operatively. Similarly, the surgeon should also be careful in looking into all angles of possible complications for given individual and making a correct plan and a road map for surgery.

Complications of surgery can be divided into two groups: immediate, both intra-operative and immediate post-operative, and delayed. Immediate complications could be surgery or anesthesia related. Immediate surgical complications include bleeding, hematoma, infections, etc. The delayed complications could be unsatisfactory scarring, asymmetry, wound dehiscence, etc. There are specific complications associated with specific surgery. For example, in face lift operations a patient may develop bleeding or injury to facial nerves during surgery, or may develop bleeding in the immediate post-operative period. On the other hand, the patient may develop inadequate face lift or scar formation, or hair loss, at a delayed period. Pre-operative explanation of the possible risks and complications helps the patient and doctor to cope with untoward complications in a rational way. If explained to a patient beforehand that control of pre-existing hypertension is important to avoid bleeding during or after surgery, there is a high probability the patient will take the pre-operative medications as suggested by the physician.

Learning the Skills in Order – A to Z

The best way to learn the skills of plastic surgery is to go through regular training of plastic surgery in a ACGME approved residency program.

During your learning phase, don't try to focus on only one aspect of plastic surgery; learn the broad-based skills. For example, don't focus on burns or facial or maxillary injury. Learn about skin cancer, cosmetic surgery and pediatric surgery, etc. Then modify that basic training to suite your need. Don't walk before you crawl. Avoid situations where you, figuratively, go to graduate school and then try to learn high school lessons. Learn the field from A to Z. All surgical training is graded. It is difficult to read a book from the end.

Three things are essential: technical skills, imagination, and honesty. If you are knowledgeable, imaginative, and critical, you can figure things out and be a great surgeon. Three-dimensional vision, curiosity, use of common sense and good planning are key to successful outcomes. Visualize how things will look at the end of the operation before you begin. Be self-critical, honest and mostly patient proponent.

Keeping Up to Date Technologically

If you plan to go to Australia next month, before you go you read up on what to expect in Australia, what you want to see, and plan to ask people when you get there what they suggest you see and do. You build your knowledge base.

Knowledge of medicine is a sum of cumulative education and training and is updated through books and journals and meetings. Updates also come about through conversations with people. Sometimes people do not write down information, but if you ask them, they will give you information. If you have common sense, are knowledgeable and listen, chances are you will learn as you grow in the medical field.

You should have fundamental understandings of your field, and if you are knowledgeable, you should be able to understand not only the medical aspects, but also the social history to help you see the whole picture. I try to be critical – you have to be critical. I believe reading and having an open mind is the key.

Striking a Balance: Professional and Personal Lives

English is not my first language and I discovered when I started learning English that the saying is true: "If you want to learn a language, you must eat the language, sleep the language, and dream the language." You cannot learn from merely listening. That is, if I wanted to learn English, I had to *think* in English.

In plastic surgery, or any medical field, your life truly rotates around what you want to learn. The balancing is tough. Every individual has to discover his or her own way of balancing.

A supportive family is critical for achieving balance. On the other hand there should be a separation of personal and medical life. Otherwise, work can be an ever consuming affair. My wife and I are both physicians. From day one, we decided we will not talk about medicine or work at home. Otherwise, life becomes a 24-hour medical thought process which can be tiring.

Plastic Surgery's Most Challenging Aspects

Because of the media, the money and people's expectations, the most challenging aspect of our specialty is the amount of myth generated about what we can and cannot do. The challenge is to be able to explain to a patient why cosmetic surgery is not the solution for personal and social problems. Myths like laser surgery not resulting in scars and skin grafts correcting all deformities are rampant among the lay population. These plastic surgery myths make it difficult for reasonable plastic surgeons to explain the impossibility of "no complication lunch time face lifts," "non-surgical face lifts" or "special bra induced breast augmentation" to knowledgeable patients. The challenge is to explain to the patient that something he has heard is a myth or a gimmick. I have to explain in medical terms that there are risks and benefits with anything we do. Total makeover as they see in television can be a dangerous procedure if things do not go as planned or expected. It may have its disastrous consequences. To make a patient understand what is achievable and the associated risks of any kind of surgery can be sometimes challenging and difficult.

It is also tough to keep up with technical skills. Advances in this field are faster than in practically any other specialty. One has to keep track of all the new things.

I have to make an effort to avoid being perceived as a glamorous surgeon. People's perception about plastic surgery or the surgeon can get into your head after a while, if you let it. One has to stay focused and grounded and, at the same time, stay continuously updated on the new science and technical skills that come from all over the world.

Success and Respect in the Field

You measure success in your own way. I believe success can be measured by someone else – your peers, for instance. I believe I am successful because I do things that work and I feel content about what I do. Success is dictated by whichever parameter you want to use. Some people measure it by financial gain; others by the successful outcome of a challenging case.

I am impressed by an honest and educated surgeon who has both feet on the ground. There is nothing like a brave surgeon, only the brave patient. When I listen to doctors or watch them operate, and I see they are honest, understand their mistakes and modify their actions accordingly, they become respectful physicians. Medicine is a dynamic specialty. Every disease or situation teaches something. It is only the smart doctors who learn from them – sometimes from a mistake and sometimes from a successful outcome. A respectful doctor is not a dogmatic individual. He or she is flexible and knows how to modify their plan of management as situation evolves.

Selecting the Right Plastic Surgeon

Using common sense is critical in selecting a plastic surgeon. The number one criterion is that the surgeon has to be well educated and well trained. He must have full training in plastic surgery and be board eligible or board-certified. Those are the basic criteria, but not the only ones.

The patient must also meet with the surgeon, ask questions, be doubtful, and see how he handles the situation. Can he answer the questions? If he explains things to the patient in terms which are ununderstandable medical jargons then the patient should stay away from that individual. The doctor must be able to explain things in layman's terms. Lack of basic understanding of the problem on the part of the plastic surgeon usually results in use of complex medical terminology.

The patient should ask people for references if a particular doctor has treated them.

The patient should never select a plastic surgeon on the basis of how the doctor's office looks, how his secretary looks, or whether he has gold jewelry or a stunning haircut.

I personally think patients should select from physicians at universities or residency training centers. I may be am biased, but I am a university surgeon advocate. Universities use stringent criteria to ensure physician quality because when patients go to a university hospital, there isn't just one doctor seeing patients. A large university has a massive staff, which provides quality assurance. The bad doctors are ejected from the system over time. For instance, I have two students and two residents standing next to me. Even the students and residents would know if a doctor is not honest. And within a year, everyone would know, and he or she would be dealt with.

Patients should not select a surgeon because of an ad. Publications and advertisements are important, but when a surgeon represents his practice with a picture of a half-naked female or a model to attract patients, the patients should bear in mind that they will not look like the model in the ad. A sound medical practice and a deceptive advertisement should not go hand in hand.

Word-of-mouth is the best way to settle on a doctor to perform plastic surgery.

Bad Decisions Benefit No One

I dislike seeing a well-trained plastic surgeon become a businessman with his entire thought processes focused on how to make money from his patients. It's a terrible shame when a doctor begins selling operations – for example, when a patient wants his nose done, and the surgeon thinks in terms of the $3,000 he will collect from the patient and pushes to sell him a bit of a facelift for another $4,000.

Another problem arises when a patient asks a doctor to do things that the doctor knows are not doable: "Make me look like Britney Spears." Even if the patient offers a large and tempting bonus, the surgeon must decline if he or she feels that patient has unrealistic expectations.

It is equally wrong to do surgery when you know the procedure will produce a bad outcome just to please the patient. People in distress cannot always make rational decisions. They are vulnerable. Plastic surgeons should help people in that frame of mind, guiding them to make good decisions. A classic example would be the surgeon who has operated multiple times on people like Michael Jackson. Though I am not privileged to have all the information of the surgery performed on him, it seems it would have been more useful for him to have all the consequences of the procedures and realistic outcomes known to him. And sometimes refusal to do surgery may be a better choice for some patients. We all have been victims of such situations in our career at some time in our life. Our decisions can get clouded by the sheer good intention to help a patient even when in the back of our mind we know the outcome may not be satisfactory. "Knowing when to walk away" can save the day.

Advances in the Profession

Plastic surgery has changed enormously in the last five to ten years. It is now very focused on specialties, like cosmetic surgery or craniofacial surgery, for example.

The research and activity in plastic surgery have changed. Previously, a post heart operation patient, for example, with an infection in the chest wall had a mortality rate of about 70 percent. Now we can offer these patients help that takes the mortality rate down to zero because we know how to bring in new blood supplies and how to make the wound heal faster.

There have been enormous developments in cosmetic surgery. Our earlier knowledge of regular face lifts has grown phenomenally. Now we know that just a face lift doesn't work; patients have to change their nutritional habits. We have found that simply taking out skin doesn't work; we have to bring in muscle, too. Now surgeons are open-minded enough that they accept that maybe they have to change the skin tone, as well.

Five years back, you couldn't find alpha hydroxy cream in stores. Now you can't go to stores without seeing the creams with various acids added – fruit acids and others. Scientists have figured out the importance and advantage of toning the muscles. Now we are using electrical stimulation to make muscles stronger, and we're using other new techniques, as well. In the past, if patients lost bone, they ended up having an amputation. Now we have bone substitutes and implants of various kinds.

In the past, we never used microscopes in plastic surgery. Now we use microscopes in all kinds of surgeries.

Future Developments: Such Vast Possibilities

We will discover better wound healing material, better scar modification material, and better muscle-toning mechanisms. Some of them will be discovered in non-surgical ways.

I think more and more doctors will think not just of the surgical aspect of plastic surgery, but also of using anti-aging medication and anti-aging treatments in their practices. We will see plastic surgeons in the forefront of the anti-aging medications, using hormones, exercise, exfoliative chemicals and spas to make people look and stay looking younger and function better.

The age of the population is increasing steadily. For people who make it to age 68, there is a high probability that they will live and function until they are 80 or 85. When that happens, people will also want to look reasonably good. The major trend will be the anti-aging medicine and regime.

Personally, I would like to see wounds close faster. We continuously work on various kinds of instruments and medications for faster healing time and better appearance after the wounds heal. I'd like to have available something that voids the need for skin grafts. I want to have bone substitutes available so we don't have to use real bones. And I'd like to be able to heal a fracture not by opening it and putting in a plate, but maybe by using a special type of glue that heals the fracture and makes the site look good.

The field is vast and wide open. Every day, students tell me about new ideas they have. People who say we cannot advance anymore than we have are being very shortsighted. We are limited only by our imaginations. Wound healing, anti-aging treatments, substitutes for skin and bone, and various artificial organs may be possible through stem cells. Perhaps we could learn to create a heart or a hand. All these things are possible.

My advice is that if you plan to specialize in medicine, don't do so for financial reasons, but because it interests you. Diseases must interest you; people must interest you. You must feel compelled to do something to help people. If you want to find shortcuts in life, don't go into medicine. There are no shortcuts in learning.

You must be curious. You must always ask why.

Recognized since 1994 by Philadelphia Magazine as one of the region's "Top Docs" in plastic and reconstructive surgery and also by the Consumer's Advocate Group, Amitabha (Amit) Mitra, M.D., M.S., F.R.C.S., F.A.C.S., is the Director of Hand and Microvascular Surgery, as well as professor and Chief of Plastic Surgery at Temple University Health Sciences Center. He is also Chief of Plastic Surgery at Shriner's Hospital for Children, Episcopal Hospital, and Temple Children's. Dr. Mitra graduated from the University of Calcutta with multiple honors and received his M.D. from the University Delhi in India.

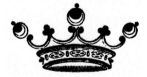

Plastic Surgery and Plastic Surgeons in the 21st Century

Khosrow Matini, M.D., FACS

Chief of Plastic Surgery, INOVA Mount Vernon Hospital; *Director*, Rejuvenation Center for Plastic Surgery

Consequence of Detail

Plastic surgery is a living compendium of the progress in the art of surgery. Refinements are constantly ongoing in the surgery of aging faces, body contouring, corrections of congenital deformities of the face, increased understanding of the etiology of wound healing and tissue transplantation, reconstruction of the face by complex craniofacial osteotomy, and others. All these together form the current state of plastic surgery.

A plastic surgeon is like a music conductor. He or she ensures harmony between the science and the art. Although the best musicians, painters, and sculptors have fantastic artistic talents, they are not able to change the face or body of a person because they lack knowledge of the science. The knowledge of the science is necessary to bring the art and beauty to reality in a human being.

Plastic surgery is not only a technical challenge, but more importantly, it is a challenge to one's aesthetic sensibility – one's ability to appreciate the consequences of minute or subtle detail. The consequence of the details is the key to great results in plastic surgery.

Plastic Surgery's Role in Treating the Whole Person

The aesthetics of plastic surgery can be divided into two parts. Aesthetic plastic surgery, though admittedly done on occasion to rehabilitate a particular part of the body, is mainly performed to rehabilitate the entire person. An individual's psyche suffers ruptures and tears paralleling that of tissue showing advancing age or the ravages of disease or injury.

In other circumstances, tissue changes result in part or in total from emotional disturbances, which may be the cause rather than the effect. It stands to reason that the improvement of the appearance of a person means his or her self-image is improved. This change, in turn, provides a feeling of emotional and physical well-being.

In addition, the plastic surgeon is called on to help other surgical specialties. The reality is that in every surgical specialty, there are circumstances where the help of the plastic surgeon is needed.

For example, if a general surgeon is removing a large cancerous tumor of the shoulder, to cure the patient, he has to remove the tumor and even some healthy tissue around it. That creates such a complex wound that it requires the expertise of a plastic surgeon for closure. This requires tissue transfer from a distance.

The same goes for Otolaryngologists who do radical resections of cancer in the head and neck region and create complex defects which require tissue transfer to reconstruct and close the defect.

In orthopedic surgery, for example, patients with open fractures of leg and soft tissue loss create a complex wound with exposure of broken bone. There is a need for plastic surgeons to cover the exposed bone of the front of the leg by a muscle from the back of the same leg. The knowledge of muscle flap reconstruction saves these injured legs today while prior to 1970 a lot of these injuries ended in amputation of the legs.

Dealing with Recent Changes

Plastic surgeons, like all other physicians, face increasing premiums for malpractice insurance. The problem has grown to the point where some doctors have had to close their offices and look for other types of work. Several well established insurance companies, like St. Paul Insurance Company and recently Farmer's Insurance Group, have stopped offering malpractice insurance. The doctors who were with them were caught off guard when the companies informed them that they wouldn't have insurance anymore. That is a big concern.

In last few years, the concept of filling the depressed region of the face, as a result of aging, has become popular. Different fillers such as fat from patients' own body collagen or from human cadaver skin or cow are used to rejuvenate the skin of the face.

Resurfacing the facial skin by laser, chemical or sanding are also helpful to stimulate the production of new collagen and rejuvenation of the face. Exfoliating products which patients can apply to their face at home on a daily basis stimulate the skin cells to produce new collagen. This is a part of the skin treatment program that I offer my patients. Repositioning of misplaced facial tissues is another new concept in rejuvenation.

Communications with Patients and the Public

The best plastic surgeons are honest, direct, and open with their patients. They should be available to answer patients' questions prior to surgery and after surgery – specifically after surgery, because the patients are worried. They should be able to spend unlimited time with patients either during the consultation or after surgery and be available to other physicians when our expertise is needed.

I try to be honest and straightforward with my patients from the beginning to the end. If a complication arises, I don't try to hide it. I inform the patient immediately and let him or her know it will be fixed. I think the direct line of communication makes the patient aware from the first consultation that I am available for them at any time.

I always return phone calls on the same day I receive them. If a patient has a concern about his or her condition after surgery, I always tell my staff that I want to see the patient the same day. That reduces the apprehension and anxiety of the patient, and at the same time, if there is a problem early recognition and treatment will improve the final outcome. Also the patient sees that I truly care about them.

I conduct frequent seminars on plastic surgery for physicians and the public. I can talk to them in a different way. People register to attend a seminar in which I talk about different subjects, not just cosmetic surgery. I talk about skin cancer and protection of the skin from the sun. I talk to them about the non-surgical modalities available for the aging face, as well as the surgical techniques available for rejuvenation. The people who attend the meetings can ask me practically anything. I have found this open communication to be very helpful for the public.

Making Decisions and Treatment Plans

When patients usually make appointments for consultations, they will say what the reason for the consultation is. Therefore, when the patient arrives in the office for aesthetic surgery consultation, my staff knows what procedure the patient is seeking for consult. The patient will be taken to a room to watch a video related to the procedure. Then I will talk to the patient and examine them. I suggest the best procedure that will improve their condition. I also talk to them about the alternative procedures, the possibility of permanent scarring, expected results, the course of convalescence and possible complications. Then I show them photographs of previous patients who have had similar surgeries. If necessary, I draw schematic pictures. Before they leave the consultation room, I remind them if they or their family have any further questions, I will be glad to answer them.

I do all my surgeries in the hospital, either as outpatient or inpatient. I believe the hospital is a safer environment for surgery.

When patients make their decision for surgery, my nurse makes them a preoperative appointment approximately two weeks prior to surgery. At the time of this appointment, the patients read a comprehensive consent form which has been prepared for each procedure and signs it. This consent form gives the patient detailed information about the surgery, alternative surgery or procedures, and a list of possible complications. It also lists the medications they should not take from that time until the day of surgery. If certain tests are necessary to be done prior to surgery, arrangements are made for them. The preoperative photograph is taken at that time. The non-aesthetic patients are treated in the same fashion.

Risks for the Plastic Surgeon

If a plastic surgeon operates on patients with unrealistic expectations, he should expect unhappy patients – no matter how successful the surgery. For instance, when a patient brings along a picture of a movie star and requests a nose or face like that picture, I tell them that is not possible. I steer away from operating on people with such requests. No matter how good of a job you do, the person will never look like the picture.

The second risk group for plastic surgeons includes those patients who want a procedure done to their body or face not because they are unhappy about it, but because they think the results will impress a boyfriend, girlfriend or spouse and make them happier.

I was very lucky. Just before I started my plastic surgery training, I saw a movie called *Ash Wednesday* about a very rich couple played by Henry Fonda and Elizabeth Taylor. They'd been married for 30 years, and the wife felt her husband was no longer interested in her, so she went to a famous clinic in Switzerland and had extensive plastic surgery done. She stayed there to recover, then called her husband to come and meet her for a few days together. The husband came, and the wife was happy – until he served her divorce papers over dinner. That movie provided a very effective lesson for me.

A mother once brought in her 15-year-old daughter and asked me to fix her daughter's nose. I asked the mother if I could speak to her daughter in her absence and in the presence of my nurse. When I talked to the daughter, she had no interest in changing the shape of her nose. Perhaps she would change her mind two or three years later, but at that point, no matter what changes I made to her nose, she would not have been happy with the result.

I deal with these kinds of situations regularly. Usually I first see the parent and child together, then I see the patient without the parent and then I talk to the parents privately. I explain to them that I understand they have good intentions in wanting to make their daughter more beautiful, but she also has to want it. If she does not want it, I explain, she will be very unhappy, no matter what I do.

Similarly, if a person is considering surgery because he or she wants to make someone else happy, it will never have a happy ending. Those are risky situations I try to avoid.

It is very difficult in the beginning of a practice, when the doctor is hungry for patients, to refuse to do a surgery, but I think if he does surgery on patients like those, he will suffer for a long time.

Sharing Expertise

I have found it effective to inform my medical and surgical colleagues about what I can do and what my expertise is, and if they ask, I talk to them about different procedures. I let them know I am available for lecturing on any subject they'd like to hear about.

I made a brochure about breast reconstruction and donated it to a general surgeon's office to put in their waiting room. The information covered who is a candidate for breast reconstruction, what is involved, different modality of breast reconstruction. It also talked about the healing process and the risks involved, and it provided a schematic drawing of each procedure, each technique..

Keeping Knowledge Fresh

Professionally, I try to read several plastic surgery journals and attend four or five national and international meetings and conventions every year. After one convention, when the planners asked what I thought of the sessions, I told them that paper presentations of five or six minutes do not teach the audience anything. In fact, they make it so that someone in the audience might think that they can just go home and start doing the procedure described in the paper without any problems. I suggested that the best way to teach surgeons new procedures and techniques is to *show* them how to do it.

Fortunately, in many meetings now, the surgeon presenting a new technique shows a video. Sometimes I attend courses where the surgeon actually performs surgery in an operating room, and we view the procedure from a conference room where we have direct contact with the surgeon and can ask questions. The surgeons can buy the videos and review them at any time, which is very helpful, especially when the procedure is one we haven't done before.

Plastic surgery is evolving so fast. When I finished my training in 1976, there was no muscle surgery. I took a seven-day workshop about muscle flaps and performed every new muscle flap surgery on a cadaver in an anatomy lab. Sometimes I do a new procedure on a cadaver first to make sure it is workable. Then, when I meet with a patient, I tell them I haven't done this new procedure yet, but I have seen it performed with good results, and I'd like to try it. If they agree, then I do it.

Roadblocks: Seeking Help from Other Plastic Surgeons

When I am unfamiliar with a certain procedure, I consult other plastic surgeons, calling locally, nationally, and internationally. On one occasion, I had a patient with a problem that I caused. Although I knew how to fix the problem, I called another plastic surgeon whose expertise was in that region, and I sent the patient to that doctor. I paid for the trip and the surgery. The problem was corrected, and my patient was very happy.

If you really care about your patients as human beings, that is the kind of care you must give them. When I have questions, I talk to colleagues – I just pick up the phone and call someone in Paris or Switzerland. If you are still uncertain, find an expert in the field and send the patient to him or her.

We all see each other's patients. A patient who has had a procedure done by Dr. Smith, for example, and is not happy with the results may come to see me. And my patients may go to Dr. Smith.

I respect surgeons when they evaluate a patient as they would evaluate a patient they operated on themselves. They tell the patient their honest, truthful opinion. Unfortunately, when many doctors, especially the younger ones, hear complaints from patients, their first reaction when they see the patient is to blurt out, "Oh, my god!" That reaction obviously makes the patients even more upset than they were before. I respect surgeons who are honest with their own patients, as well as with other plastic surgeons' patients.

Must Haves: Honesty, Availability

My advice is to make sure you have enough knowledge for the types of surgery you choose to do. There are certain types of plastic surgery I will not do. When a patient comes to me for consultation, I tell them I am sorry, I do not do this procedure, and I refer the patient to someone who does. I don't charge for the consultation, even those cases that are covered by insurance.

In addition, be knowledgeable and honest with patients and be available to them. The biggest complaint I have heard – and I think many times this initiates a malpractice suit – is that, after surgery, patients cannot reach their doctor. They think something is wrong, or perhaps something is bothering them. They don't know what is normal the day after surgery; after all, they are patients, not plastic surgeons. They look at themselves and say, "Oh my! What have I done?"

They need the doctor to see them right away, to reassure them. Maybe it takes five or ten minutes of my time to examine them and reassure them everything is normal. Otherwise, if I don't see them, they become more and more worried. Regardless of the situation, when I hear a patient wants to see me and I do not know what the complaint may be, I become worried. In 27 years, I have been sued only once, and I won before a jury and was vindicated.

End Goal: Best Results for the Patient

The worst part of being a plastic surgeon is that we are the end of the line. Other doctors send patients to me when they are having problems, but I cannot send patients elsewhere unless, as I said, there is a field of plastic surgery I do not do. But outside that situation, I am the one to solve the problem.

I had a hand surgery fellowship in Louisville with one of the best hand surgeons in the world, Dr. Harold Kleinert, who was running that program. Dr. Kleinert used to say, "This is the Mecca of hand surgery. We cannot send patients anywhere else. We have to take care of them."

The ultimate goal is to solve the patient's problem. If I can't, I consult other plastic surgeons. If they say they would like to see the patient, then I refer the patient to them. If the patient was operated on by me, I always ask the surgeon not to charge the patient, and if there is a charge, to please send the bill to me.

The bottom line is that the patient should receive the best results. Even if in the middle of surgery I have a problem, I call someone else to come and look over me. I don't have the kind of ego that makes me believe I am a god and no one else knows anything. I have no qualms about asking nurses and anesthesiologists – the people working with me in surgery – how the results look to them. If someone says it looks like this one is a little smaller or larger than that one, I don't get upset; I appreciate their candor. The more successful the surgery, the better for the patient and for me.

From Good to Great: Caring Personally and Professionally

Many people believe a plastic surgeon's mission is to write a lot of papers, and that's what makes great plastic surgeons. I think great plastic surgeons are remembered by their patients for other reasons.

I care about people personally, and I care immensely about my patients professionally. During difficult situations, when it is tough to make a decision about a patient, I always imagine the patient is my sister, my mother, or my brother. What would I want for them if they were in the same situation or had the same condition? That helps me make the right decision because I know I would not make a bad decision for a family member.

I can remember many cases where I have seen happiness in the faces of the parents or the patients, and I will never forget that.

I recall an 18-year-old girl who had been born with a cleft lip that had been repaired, and the family was not happy with the result. Now she was growing, and her upper lip was tight, so they brought her to me. She was a very attractive young lady. I reconstructed her upper lip deficiency by moving a portion of the lower lip up. For about ten days, her upper and lower lips were sewn together. After the second stage, when we divided the lips and put them back together, I came to the recovery room to talk to the parents. I had never met her father before, just her mother. Her father, an army captain, said, "Dr.

Matini, I heard that you have a daughter too. You must know how happy I am looking at the face of my daughter for the first time like this."

I operated on a five-year-old from a third-world country. No one could determine why she couldn't open her mouth. She was being fed through tubes and with a tiny, tiny spoon. The X-ray and the tomogram we took showed that both joints of the jaw were fused. Probably when she was a baby, she fell and broke her jaw, and no one recognized that one side had fused. When I operated on her, I created new joints on both sides. Two days after surgery, she was able to open her mouth. I will never forget the happiness on the faces of her parents. And I am sure they will never forget me.

These are the kinds of things that make a plastic surgeon – or a journalist or an ambulance driver – great; they create happiness in others.

Try, Try Again

I believe plastic surgeons should have multiple armaments in their skills bag. When one approach doesn't work, they find another way to solve the problem.

When I was in training, and later, when attending meetings, I heard this advice over and over: In plastic surgery there is no one way to perform a particular operation for every case. The procedure must be adaptable, and the surgeon must be inventive in applying basic knowledge of aesthetics together with the science and the art of plastic surgery.

The golden rule for plastic surgery is planning and having multiple plans in mind. If plan A is not working, the doctor can use plan B. Do not break bridges before you make a new bridge. If plan A doesn't work and you have not destroyed the possibility of plan B working, you are okay. But if you think plan A is definitely working and cut the tissue that could be used for plan B, when plan A doesn't work, you are stuck. It is important to have contingency plans in your mind when you go into the operating room. After a while, it becomes automatic, and you don't have to think about it.

For example, I scheduled a patient far in advance for a face lift and eyelid surgery. The patient had been on blood thinners. After consulting her cardiologist, we asked her not to take the blood thinner medication four days prior to surgery. She came to the holding area before we began surgery on her, we repeated her blood test, and her blood was still thin. We had to tell the patient we couldn't operate on her. The patient was disappointed, the husband was disappointed, and I lost five hours of operating room time, but there was no other way if we wanted to do a safe surgery. We rescheduled the same patient and when she came to the holding area of the operating room, we checked her blood pressure; it was too high, even though earlier in my office her blood pressure had been normal. But I had to tell her again that I couldn't operate on her. When we scheduled this woman for the third time, two days before surgery she fell and injured her face and her face lift surgery was cancelled. We never did do surgery on her!

These are not easy decisions to make because there are many financial repercussions. The patient might even change her mind. But I am happy I didn't operate because if I had, at any of those stages, I would have faced multiple complications and problems.

Emerging Techniques and Practices

In the next five years, I believe there will be new technology for creating new techniques for different problems, and new fillers will come to the market. We have been using fillers for the last few years while we try to find fillers that stay in the body for a long time – even for good. The body absorbs most fillers after a few months. The only one we have that stays for good is fat that belongs to the patient.

I also believe that in the next five years, the new horizon for plastic surgery will be bariatric plastic surgery, which is cosmetic plastic surgery for more than one area of the body. Those areas may include the face, neck, chest, breast, arms, abdominal wall, back, and thighs. It is used frequently after a massive loss of body weight, as a result of bariatric surgery.

We have about 40 million obese patients in this country, and 8 million of them are morbidly obese. With this new surgical approach of a duodenal switch or gastric bypass, the patients lose 100 to 150 pounds. The obesity is corrected, which eases the burden on the patients' hearts, and their blood pressure improves, but they look terrible because of the pendulous skin. A 30-year-old body looks like an 85-year-old body. Everything hangs.

This is a very challenging field that will grow tremendously. In 2003, probably 70,000 people had this type of operation. Each stage of surgery is a long operation and a multi-stage operation is needed because you can't fix the whole body in one sitting. The body contouring surgery after bariatric surgery requires multiple stages of surgery averaging five to seven hours long. The average cost of total facial and body contouring is around $70000.00. This, of course, includes the surgeon fee, anesthesiologist fee, and hospital cost.

I believe that embryonic tissue research will expand. This type of tissue will be used to treat many diseases and problems we cannot treat today. And gene therapy, which has already begun, will expand in the next five years.

Hope for the Future: Controlling the Problem of Scarring

When I was in high school, I had a teacher for composition who one day gave us this topic: If you were a creator, how would you create your creature? I will never forget what I wrote and what I am faced with today.

If I could create a drug, it would be a drug to control scarring and promote healing. Uncontrolled and undesirable scarring causes many medical and surgical problems and diseases. Somebody gets an infection in the kidney. The body tries to fight the infection, and the result is that eventually that area where the body is fighting the infection heals and creates scar tissue. Unfortunately, we have no control over how much the scar tissue grows. It can grow to the point that it starts to choke the rest of the good tissue of the kidney. That is why, from a medical standpoint, there is no treatment available for kidney disease today and this has not changed.

During the last five hundred years they did not have the technology we have today. When someone's kidney didn't work, we put them on dialysis, and today we have technology that finds a kidney to match the patient's for a transplant. But we have not been able to treat liver disease, kidney disease, nerve disease, and other conditions caused by scarring. If someone gets hepatitis, the part of the liver shows the damage and fills up with scar tissue. Sometimes the scar tissue grows so large that it chokes the rest of the liver, causing cirrhosis, and the patient loses the function of the liver.

If we could find a medication to use for different stages of healing and on different types of tissue, we could then control the healing process and scarring, but prevent further formation of scarring when it begins to damage the tissue. For that, we need more than one plastic surgeon. We need a team of biochemists, pharmaceutical experts, inventors – and plastic surgeons. There has been a great deal of work on wound healing, which is why some progress has been evident in tissue transplants. Still though, we are far from where we need to be to resolve the issue of scar damage.

Some medications already available can control certain scarring, but they have so many side effects that we cannot use them. The ideal environment for surgery is fetal. When we perform surgery on a fetus inside the mother's body, our cutting and sewing does not leave scars. Discovering how to get to that condition in the rest of us will probably happen at some point.

There is major controversy about using the placenta tissue or new tissue for research studies when the baby is aborted. That tissue can be used to make anything out of it. In the adult form of the human body, only liver cells and the top layer of the skin can regenerate. The rest of the body cannot regenerate, so we borrow skin from another part of the body to cover the area. The cells for making a new baby can form bone, marrow, blood vessels, and skin. I think that is where research will go in the future.

Founder and director of the Rejuvenation Center for Plastic Surgery, Dr. Khosrow Matini is Chief of Plastic Surgery and a past-president of the medical staff at INOVA Mount Vernon Hospital. He has served INOVA Mount Vernon Hospital in many capacities, including Chairman of the Department of Surgery from 1989 to 1990. Dr.

Matini also holds privileges as a member of the Department of Surgery at INOVA Alexandria and INOVA Fairfax hospitals.

Born in Tehran, Iran, Dr. Matini obtained his medical degree with distinction from the Meshed University School of Medicine in 1966, followed by an internship at Providence Hospital in Washington D.C. After completing four years of general surgery training at the Jewish Hospital Medical Center of New York, and the University of Louisville, Kentucky, he obtained a fellowship in hand surgery at the latter. Dr. Matini then completed two years of residency in Plastic and Reconstructive Surgery at George Washington University, where he then went on to serve as Assistant Clinical Professor of Plastic and Reconstructive Surgery (1976-1978) before entering private practice in Virginia.

Dr. Matini is Board Certified by the American Board of Surgery, and the American Board of Plastic Surgery – the only board for plastic surgery recognized by the American Board of Medical Specialties.

Dr. Matini served as President of the Alexandria Medical Society between 1996 and 1997, and is an active member of the American Society of Plastic Surgery, The American Society of Aesthetic Plastic Surgery, the American College of Surgeons, the Capital Society of Plastic Surgeons, the Virginia Medical Society, and the International Society of Aesthetic Plastic Surgeons.

Dr. Matini has been in practice in the local community for over 27 years and has performed thousands of operations, and is a leading authority on breast surgery, body contouring and aesthetic facial surgery. He is recognized as one of the Washington area's leading cosmetic plastic and reconstructive surgeons, and his experience and expertise have earned him the title of top plastic surgeon in the area by Washingtonian Magazine since 1994.

Plastic Surgery Following Bariatric Surgery

Khosrow Matini, M.D., FACS
DonnaRose Klemovitch-Rhoads, P.A.-C

The Centers for Disease Control and Prevention reported that in 2000 over 31 percent of the general population in the United States are obese. Of this figure, over 4 million people can be classified as morbidly obese, i.e. 100 or more pounds over a healthy weight. A recent study by the Rand Institute reported morbid obesity increased from 1 in 200 persons in 1986 to 1 in 50 persons in 2000.

Traditional methods of weight reduction through diet have not proven effective for the morbidly obese patient, with an average 95 percent failure rate. However, advances in bariatric surgery, with a reduction in post operative complications and morbidity, have allowed it to become a major tool for patients seeking permanent and large quantity weight reduction. It is estimated that over 100,000 bariatric surgeries will be performed in the United States in 2003.

Bariatric surgery has its own set of outcomes differing from those of a "normal" weight loss patient. One year after bariatric surgery, the average patient loses about 110 lbs. Significant weight loss leaves the bariatric surgery patient seeking body contouring procedures. Many bariatric surgery patients did not even consider the effect massive weight loss would have on their bodies; they only knew weight loss was imperative, often for health reasons.

While the average body contouring patient generally focuses on one problem area of the body requiring one or two procedures for correction, the bariatric surgery patient must deal with unacceptable appearances in multiple areas requiring extensive multiple procedures such as facial and cervical rhytidectomy, mastopexy, excision of redundant skin and subcutaneous tissues of the axilla and anterolateral aspect of the chest wall and upper back, brachioplasty, abdominoplasty, pubic mount reduction and lift, circumferential thigh lift, and buttock lift for correction. The amount of loose and hanging skin not only presents a gross unacceptable cosmetic appearance but can also result in health issues ranging from skin irritation under the hanging skin to postural changes from the weight of the hanging tissues.

In my experience, these post-bariatric patients will need more extensive surgery than the procedures they initially elect to have performed. Often, so many procedures need to be performed they will need to be accomplished in multiple phases, spaced weeks to months apart. These patients also often have a different set of expectations as to the amount of remaining scarring that that they consider acceptable and the percent of improvement in the final result. Additionally, procedures performed in the traditional, minimal scar manner, such as thigh lift and abdominoplasty, do not allow for removal of the extensive amount of skin and subcutaneous tissue present in the bariatric patient. The need for this extensive removal of tissue has challenged my surgical expertise and resulted in the use of non-traditional procedures such as inverted t-abdominoplasty with abdominal wall muscle tightening, a V-type thigh lift from the inner aspect of the knees up to the groin, and extended arm lifts requiring excision of excessive skin of the axilla, anterolateral chest wall and upper back. Many of these patients also have a ptotic pubic mount that requires reduction and/or lift.

Body Contouring Techniques Following a Major Weight Loss

Augmentation Mammoplasty and Mastopexy:

More than 90 percent of bariatric surgery patients will require augmentation mammoplasty due of the loss of volume of the breast tissue following major weight loss. Because of the severity of ptosis, in these patients submammary augmentation is preferable to subpectoral augmentation. Mastopexy should also be done following the augmentation mammoplasty at the same sitting. After the augmentation portion of the procedure is completed, the patient should be placed into the semi-sitting position on the operating table and measurements taken for lifting of the nipple areola complex. The nipple areola complex should then be moved up and the excess loose skin removed.

While many patients believe their only desire is to have their breasts lifted, once the mastopexy procedure has actually been carried out they become aware that the volume of the breasts does not match the proportions of the rest of their body and they return for augmentation. It is the duty of the plastic surgeon to advise and educate the patient prior to performing surgery that augmentation mammoplasty is necessary in the majority of bariatric surgery patients in addition to the mastopexy. The scar will be placed around the new location of the areola and between the inferior portion of the areola and the inframammary line.

During the pre-operative consultation I find the best way to determine the appropriate size of implants to use is to have the patient place different sizes of implants between their bra and breast tissue and observe themselves in a mirror wearing a form fitting top. The patient can best determine the extent of enlargement with which they feel most comfortable.

Excision of excessive skin and subcutaneous tissue of the axilla, anterolateral aspect of the chest wall, and posterior chest wall:

I have found this procedure is necessary on almost every patient who has lost more than 80 pounds following bariatric surgery. Of course, the deformity will be even more prominent on those individuals who have lost 120 to 160 pounds. This procedure involves the excision of the excessive skin of the arm pit and the excessive tissue of the lateral aspect of the chest and posterior aspect of the chest. (Figures 1, 2, 3) The surgical scar will follow the lateral portion of the breast with extension to the axilla. This procedure is necessary to achieve a nice contour of the chest, breast, axilla and goes along with the arm lift or brachioplasty.

Arm Lift (Brachioplasty):

Excision of the excessive skin and subcutaneous tissues of the inner aspect of the arm is necessary to contour the arm and get rid of the unsightly hanging tissue of the arm. Although this procedure leaves a permanent scar on the underside of the arm, the vast improvement achieved in the shape and contour of the arm justifies the permanent, visible scar.

Abdominoplasty:

The standard, hip to hip incision, type of abdominoplasty is not adequate for contouring of the abdominal wall following major weight loss. These patients have both a weakness of the abdominal wall and separation of the rectus muscle in the front of the abdomen. Therefore, they require not only removal of the excess skin and subcutaneous tissue between the umbilicus and the suprapubic area but they also require removal of the excess skin and subcutaneous tissue from the upper portion of the abdomen. (Figures 4, 5, 6) I have found the best method for this is an Inverted T-type incision. Extensive muscle tightening work also has to be performed in order to achieve further improvement of the contour of the abdomen.

Correction or improvement of the ptosis of the pubic mount:

After major weight loss the patient will most often have excess loose skin and subcutaneous tissue of the pubic mount associated with ptosis and hanging of those tissues. Therefore, at the time of the abdominoplasty, we often excise the excessive loose skin and subcutaneous tissue of the pubic mount and at the same time lift the sagging pubic mount through a V-shaped incision back to the normal position.

Inner thigh lift:

The majority of the patients, around 90 percent, will not get a good result from just a routine type of the inner thigh lift with the incision made in the groin area. A better result can be achieved with wide excision of the excess loose skin from the inner aspect of the knee and thigh all the way up to the groin area. This necessitates a V-shape incision starting from the inner aspect of the knee and ending up in the groin area. (Figures 7, 8) Though this procedure leaves a permanent scar in the inner aspect of the thigh and knee, it produces a more normal, cylindrical type of thigh shape. During this procedure the surgeon has to be careful to save the superficial venous system of the thigh.

Outer thigh lift and buttock lift:

The high weight loss patient has a tremendous sagging of the buttock along with loose skin and subcutaneous fat of the outer portion of the thighs. Excision of the excess skin above the buttock area as well as the lifting and elevation of the buttocks and outer thigh is required for correction. This procedure leaves a horizontal scar right above the buttock; however, it will be hidden nicely under a bathing suit. This operation can be performed at the same time as an inner thigh lift or it can be performed separately. This procedure also improves some of the redundancy of the skin and subcutaneous tissue of the lower back.

Facial and cervical rhytidectomy:

Many younger patients will not require facial and cervical rhytidectomy following major weight loss. However, most of the middle-aged patients will require a neck lift and some of them will require both a neck and face lift at the same time. The older patients will all require facial and cervical rhytidectomy. The technical aspects of the facial and cervical rhytidectomy in the weight loss patient is no different than that used in regular patients desiring face and neck lift for cosmetic correction of aging.

No matter what combination of procedures is performed, the post operative course for bariatric surgery patients requires longer and more labor intensive follow up and may often require coordination with various other medical specialists, such as internal medicine, endocrinology, infectious diseases and dietitians. Because of complex health issues, the time between procedures may need to be extended. This results in the plastic surgeon performing an increased role in monitoring, treating and coordinating care for multiple medical issues. The majority of these patients are anemic with low levels of serum albumin and abnormal albumin/globulin ratios. Many of them have elevation of alkaline phosphate. Many bariatric patients are diabetic or insulin resistant. They can often not tolerate blood loss during surgery and many require cc for cc blood replacement. Development of lymph collection in the medial aspect of the knee and lower thigh is common after inner thigh lift, occurring in approximately 15 percent of my patients.

The result after body contouring operations using these extensive, non-traditional techniques is striking for patients and the plastic surgeon. To see a body that appears to be 85-years old reappear to its 35-year-old actual age is a true example of the art of plastic surgery. (Figures 9, 10, 11, 12, 13, 14, 15, 16)

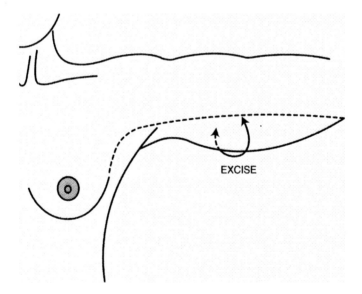

Figure 1: Location of the incision for extended armlift including excision of the excess skin of the chest and axilla.

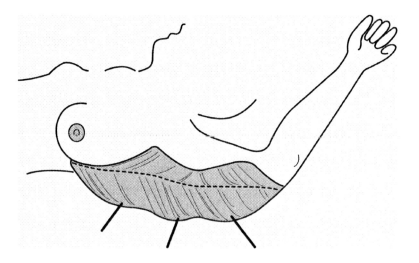

Figure 2: Schematic view of the raised skin and subcutaneous tissue flap.

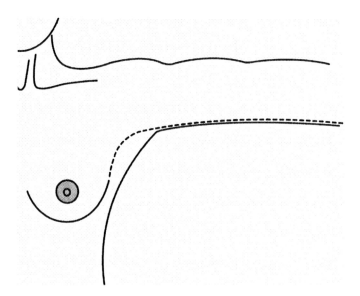

Figure 3: Location of the post operative scar after extended armlift procedure.

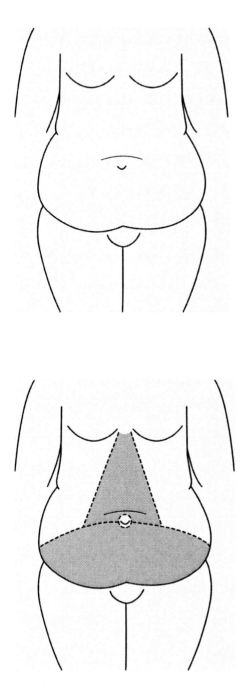

Figure 4: Schematic appearance of the abdomen following major weight loss.

Figure 5: Schematic of the location of the incisions for the inverted "T" abdominoplasty and pubic mount lift.

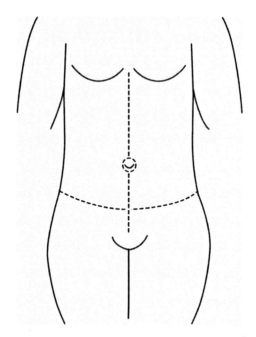

Figure 6: Schematic of the resultant scar following inverted "T" abdominoplasty and pubic mount lift.

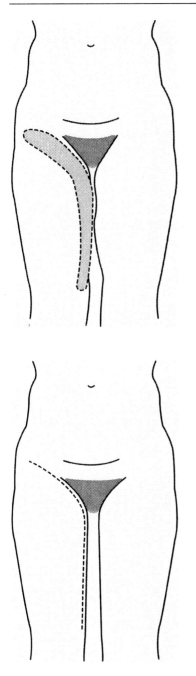

Figure 7: Schematic of location of the incisions for a "V" shaped inner thigh lift.

Figure 8: Schematic of the resultant scar following a "V" shaped inner thigh lift.

191

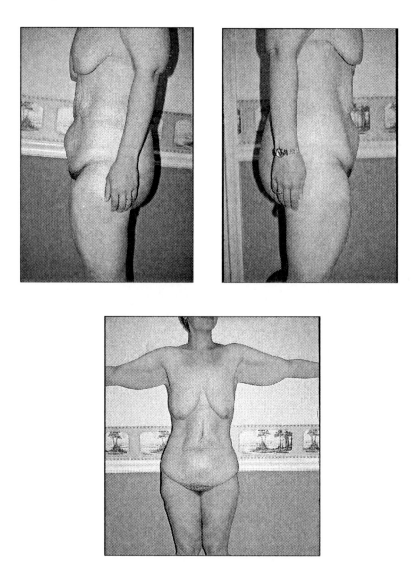

Figures 9, 10, 11: Pre-operative photographs of a 30 year old white female following 162 lbs weight loss.

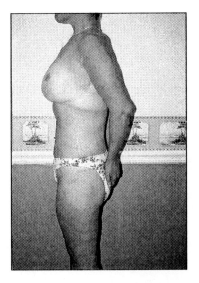 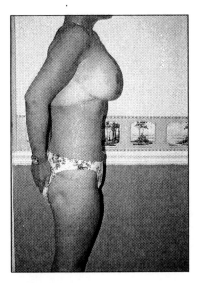

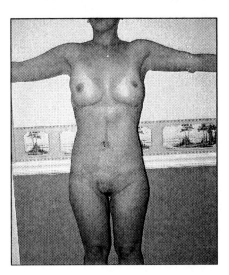

Figures 12, 13, 14: Post-operative photographs of same patient following bilateral extended armlift, mastopexy, augmentation mammoplasty, inverted "T" abdominoplasty, circumferential thigh lift, and buttock lift.

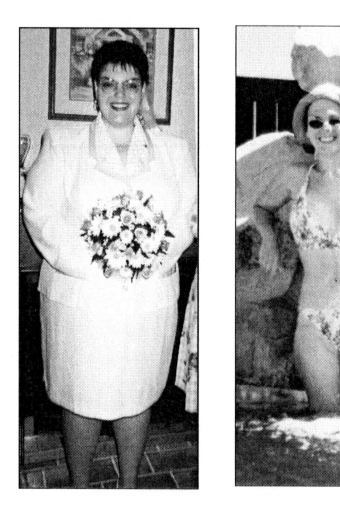

Figures 15, 16: Photographs of the same patient following 162lbs weight loss and total body contouring.

Inside the Minds:
The Art & Science of Being a Doctor
*Leading Doctors Reveal the Secrets to Professional
and Personal Success as a Doctor*

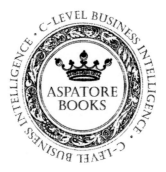

Inside the Minds: The Art & Science of Being a Doctor is the most authoritative book ever written on the medical profession, written by an unprecedented collection of leading doctors. These leading doctors reveal the secrets to patient relationships, balancing professional and personal lives, increasing your worth as a doctor, continuing research and education, time management, compensation and more. Topics also include the everlasting effects of the Internet and technology, the changing health care world, liability issues, government intervention and other important topics for all types of doctors and medical professionals. An unprecedented look inside the minds of the world's best doctors makes for critical reading for every doctor, nurse, medical student and anyone interested in the medical profession on a personal or professional level.

$37.95 – 230 Pages

Other Best Sellers

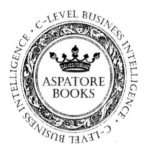